T0226375

Diffuse Gastric Cancer

Tiago Biachi de Castria
Rodrigo Santa Cruz Guindalini

Editors

Diffuse Gastric Cancer

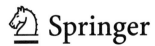 Springer

Editors
Tiago Biachi de Castria
Instituto do Câncer do Estado de São Paulo
São Paulo, São Paulo, Brazil

Rodrigo Santa Cruz Guindalini
CLION
Salvador, Bahia, Brazil

ISBN 978-3-319-95233-8   ISBN 978-3-319-95234-5   (eBook)
https://doi.org/10.1007/978-3-319-95234-5

Library of Congress Control Number: 2018954647

This Springer imprint is published by the registered company Springer Nature Switzerland AG.
The registered company address is: Gewerbestrasse 11, 6330 Cham, Switzerland

Acknowledgments

A moment of great satisfaction like this is also a moment to thank.
I would like to thank...

my family for their comprehension and love,
my teachers for serving as an example,
my patients for their daily teaching on overcoming, and
Gabriela, my wife and my safe harbor, for her unconditional support.

– Tiago Biachi de Castria

A project of this scope would not have been brought to fruition without a lot of support.

First, I would like to thank the authors of the respective chapters in this book for all their efforts, invaluable insights, and collaboration.

None of this would have been possible without my family, who has stood by me during every struggle and celebrated all my successes. A heartfelt thank you to my awesome wife, Fernanda, and my beloved daughter, Julia, for supporting and encouraging me to believe in myself and pursue my dreams.

I must express my gratitude to my teachers/mentors for their guidance, supervision, inspiration, and constructive criticism.

I am deeply indebted to my patients, who have taught me through their responses to life's daily challenges, how to become not only a better doctor but also a better human being.

Finally, I would like to thank the team at Springer for its editorial assistance.

– Rodrigo Santa Cruz Guindalini

Contents

Contributors

Paulo Pimentel de Assumpção Núcleo de Pesquisas em Oncologia, Hospital Universitário João de Barros Barreto, Universidade Federal do Pará, Guamá, Belém, Pará, Brazil

Williams Fernandes Barra Núcleo de Pesquisas em Oncologia, Hospital Universitário João de Barros Barreto, Universidade Federal do Pará, Guamá, Belém, Pará, Brazil

Tiago Biachi de Castria Instituto do Câncer do Estado de São Paulo, São Paulo, SP, Brazil

Andre Tsin Chih Chen Instituto do Câncer do Estado de São Paulo, São Paulo, SP, Brazil

Marina Candido Visontai Cormedi Faculdade de Medicina FMUSP, Universidade de Sao Paulo, Sao Paulo, SP, Brazil

Samia Demachki Núcleo de Pesquisas em Oncologia, Hospital Universitário João de Barros Barreto, Universidade Federal do Pará, Guamá, Belém, Pará, Brazil

Maria Aparecida Azevedo Koike Folgueira Faculdade de Medicina FMUSP, Universidade de Sao Paulo, Sao Paulo, SP, Brazil

Ana Carolina Ribeiro Chaves de Gouvea Centro de Oncologia Hospital Alemao Oswaldo Cruz, São Paulo, SP, Brazil

Rodrigo Santa Cruz Guindalini Centro de Investigação Translacional em Oncologia, Instituto do Câncer do Estado de São Paulo, Faculdade de Medicina da Universidade de São Paulo, São Paulo, SP, Brazil

CLION, CAM Group, Salvador, Brazil

Carlos Bo Chur Hong Faculdade de Medicina da Universidade de São Paulo/ Instituto do Câncer do Estado de São Paulo, São Paulo, SP, Brazil

Geraldo Ishak Núcleo de Pesquisas em Oncologia, Hospital Universitário João de Barros Barreto, Universidade Federal do Pará, Guamá, Belém, Pará, Brazi

Maria Lucia Hirata Katayama Faculdade de Medicina FMUSP, Universidade de Sao Paulo, Sao Paulo, SP, BR

Bruno da Costa Martins Faculdade de Medicina da Universidade de São Paulo/ Instituto do Câncer do Estado de São Paulo, São Paulo, BA, Brazil

Bruno Frederico Medrado Endoscopy section of Hospital da Clínicas, Faculdade de Medicina da Universidade Federal da Bahia, Salvador, BA, Brazil

Elizabeth Zambrano Mendoza Faculdade de Medicina da Universidade de São Paulo/Instituto do Câncer do Estado de São Paulo, São Paulo, SP, Brazil

José Mauricio Mota Instituto do Câncer do Estado de São Paulo, São Paulo, SP, Brazil

Mirella Nardo Faculdade de Medicina da Universidade de São Paulo/Instituto do Câncer do Estado de São Paulo, São Paulo, SP, Brazil

Guilherme Luiz Stelko Pereira Centro de Oncologia do Paraná, Curitiba, Paraná, Brazil

Fernando Simionato Perrotta Department of Gastroenterology, University of São Paulo School of Medicine, São Paulo, SP, Brazil

Ulysses Ribeiro Jr University of São Paulo School of Medicine, Instituto do Câncer do Estado de São Paulo, ICESP-HCFMUSP, São Paulo, SP, Brazil

Eduardo Saadi Neto Hospital de Base da Faculdade de Medicina de São José do Rio Preto (FAMERP), São José do Rio Preto, SP, Brazil

Daniela Marques Saccaro Faculdade de Medicina FMUSP, Universidade de Sao Paulo, Sao Paulo, SP, Brazil

Andrea Clemente Baptista Silva Faculdade de Medicina da Universidade de São Paulo/Instituto do Câncer do Estado de São Paulo, São Paulo, SP, Brazil

Carolina Ribeiro Victor Faculdade de Medicina da Universidade de São Paulo/ Instituto do Câncer do Estado de São Paulo, São Paulo, SP, Brazil

Chapter 1
Introduction

Tiago Biachi de Castria and José Mauricio Mota

In 1965, Laurén introduced a classification that would continue to prove its value many decades later. He recognized the existence of two major subtypes of gastric cancer: intestinal and diffuse [1]. This classification reveals profound differences in carcinogenesis, epidemiology, risk factors, molecular characteristics, prognosis, and, possibly, response to treatment. Diffuse-type adenocarcinomas have a number of special features that distinguish them from intestinal-type gastric adenocarcinomas.

Histologically, diffuse carcinomas show a lack of gland formation and less intercellular cohesion, leading to the detection of scattered small clusters of cells infiltrating the stroma, spatially separated from the primary tumor. These cells may or may not contain abundant cytoplasmic mucin producing the classic aspect of signet-ring cell. Laurén's diffuse subtype includes signet-ring cell carcinoma, which was also included in various histologic classifications, such as undifferentiated type by Nakamura in 1968 [2], infiltrative type by Ming in 1977 [3], and high grade by the American Joint Committee on Cancer/Union for International Cancer Control in 2010 [4].

Despite a progressive reduction in gastric cancer incidence and mortality, recent decades have witnessed a steady increase in the incidence of signet-ring cell gastric cancer from 0.3 cases per 100,000 persons in 1973 to 1.8 cases per 100,000 persons in 2000 in the USA [5]. Diffuse subtype is more often diagnosed at younger ages and is more evenly distributed between the sexes [6, 7].

Patients with Laurén's diffuse gastric adenocarcinoma have a worse prognosis. Locoregional disease has shown increased risk of distant recurrence and peritoneal spread [8–11]. Furthermore, gastric cancer patients with advanced disease and diffuse subtype showed reduced overall survival in a recent meta-analysis [11].

In contrast to intestinal-type gastric adenocarcinoma, the diffuse subtype is less linked to environmental factors usually associated with multistep carcinogenesis,

T. B. de Castria (✉) · J. M. Mota
Instituto do Câncer do Estado de São Paulo, São Paulo, SP, Brazil

© Springer International Publishing AG, part of Springer Nature 2018
T. B. de Castria, R. S. C. Guindalini (eds.), *Diffuse Gastric Cancer*,
https://doi.org/10.1007/978-3-319-95234-5_1

1

and precancerous lesions have not been identified. On the other hand, there is a strong association between diffuse gastric adenocarcinoma and hereditary diffuse gastric syndrome due to germline mutations in the cancer-predisposing gene *CDH1* [12]. At the molecular level, hereditary or sporadic diffuse gastric cancer usually shows a lack of E-cadherin expression or other adhesion molecules, although association with *Helicobacter pylori* has also been detected [13]. The frequency of microsatellite instability, CDX2, and HER2 expression is reduced in diffuse gastric cancer in comparison to the intestinal-type subtype [14–16].

These molecular differences may have implications for personalized treatment strategies, although the appropriate design of a tailored approach remains under investigation. The present book will present detailed, current, state-of-the-art knowledge on diffuse gastric cancer, shedding light on its epidemiology, molecular characteristics, diagnosis, and surveillance and discuss appropriate treatment for affected patients. However, the science of many of these aspects is still evolving, and much remains to be discovered that will improve the care of patients suffering from diffuse gastric cancer.

References

1. Lauren P. The two histological main types of gastric carcinoma: diffuse and so-called intestinal-type carcinoma. An attempt at a histo-clinical classification. Acta Pathol Microbiol Scand. 1965;64:31–49.
2. Nakamura K, Sugano H, Takagi K. Carcinoma of the stomach in incipient phase: its histogenesis and histological appearances. Gan. 1968;59:251–8.
3. Ming SC. Gastric carcinoma. A pathobiological classification. Cancer. 1977;39:2475–85.
4. Edge S, Byrd D, Compton C. AJCC (American Joint Committee on Cancer) cancer staging manual. 7th ed. New York: Springer; 2010.
5. Henson DE, Dittus C, Younes M, Nguyen H, Albores-Saavedra J. Differential trends in the intestinal and diffuse types of gastric carcinoma in the United States, 1973–2000: increase in the signet ring cell type. Arch Pathol Lab Med. 2004;128:765–70.
6. Correa P, Sasano N, Stemmermann GN, Haenszel W. Pathology of gastric carcinoma in Japanese populations: comparisons between Miyagi prefecture, Japan, and Hawaii. J Natl Cancer Inst. 1973;51:1449–59.
7. Piazuelo MB, Correa P. Gastric cancer: overview. Colomb Medica (Cali, Colomb). 2013;44:192–201.
8. Lee JH, Chang KK, Yoon C, Tang LH, Strong VE, Yoon SS. Lauren histologic type is the most important factor associated with pattern of recurrence following resection of gastric adenocarcinoma. Ann Surg. 2018;267:105–13.
9. Chen Y-C, Fang W-L, Wang R-F, Liu C-A, Yang M-H, Lo S-S, et al. Clinicopathological variation of Lauren classification in gastric cancer. Pathol Oncol Res. 2016;22:197–202.
10. Qiu M, Cai M, Zhang D, Wang Z, Wang D, Li Y, et al. Clinicopathological characteristics and prognostic analysis of Lauren classification in gastric adenocarcinoma in China. J Transl Med. 2013;11:58.
11. Stiekema J, Cats A, Kuijpers A, van Coevorden F, Boot H, Jansen EPM, et al. Surgical treatment results of intestinal and diffuse type gastric cancer. Implications for a differentiated therapeutic approach? Eur J Surg Oncol. 2013;39:686–93.

12. Yakirevich E, Resnick MB. Pathology of gastric cancer and its precursor lesions. Gastroenterol Clin North Am. 2013;42:261–84.
13. Palestro G, Pellicano R, Fronda GR, Valente G, De Giuli M, Soldati T, et al. Prevalence of Helicobacter pylori infection and intestinal metaplasia in subjects who had undergone surgery for gastric adenocarcinoma in Northwest Italy. World J Gastroenterol. 2005;11:7131–5.
14. Il PD, Yun JW, Park JH, Oh SJ, Kim HJ, Cho YK, et al. HER-2/neu amplification is an independent prognostic factor in gastric cancer. Dig Dis Sci. 2006;51:1371–9.
15. Almeida R, Almeida J, Shoshkes M, Mendes N, Mesquita P, Silva E, et al. OCT-1 is overexpressed in intestinal metaplasia and intestinal gastric carcinomas and binds to, but does not transactivate, CDX2 in gastric cells. J Pathol. 2005;207:396–401.
16. Kim H, An JY, Noh SH, Shin SK, Lee YC, Kim H. High microsatellite instability predicts good prognosis in intestinal-type gastric cancers. J Gastroenterol Hepatol. 2011;26:585–92.

Chapter 2
Epidemiology

Williams Fernandes Barra, Samia Demachki, Geraldo Ishak, and Paulo Pimentel de Assumpção

Incidence and Mortality

Gastric cancer, with 984,000 new cases and 841,000 deaths estimated to have occurred in 2013, is the fifth most common malignancy and the second leading cause of cancer death worldwide [1]. This disease used to be the leading cause of cancer deaths until 1980s, when it was exceeded by lung cancer [2].

Approximately 80–90% of gastric carcinomas develop in a sporadic setting, and the remaining show familial clustering, with approximately 1–3% exhibiting a clear inherited genetic susceptibility [3].

Worldwide, both the incidence of the disease and overall survival rates vary significantly. Incidence is strongly affected by ethnic and geographical factors: it is higher in Eastern Asia, Eastern Europe, and South America, while North America and Africa show the lowest rates [1, 4].

Recent decades have seen a progressive reduction in the incidence of gastric cancer across the globe (Fig. 2.1) [1]. This reduction began in those countries that had the lowest rate, while the decline rate is lower in countries with higher incidences [1]. Distal cancer (antrum and pylorus) are more common in high-incidence and high-mortality areas, and the incidence of this type of gastric cancer has decreased significantly [5]. This trend is attributed to the knowledge and control of risk factors such as *Helicobacter pylori* and other dietary and environmental factors [1]. In the USA, from 1977 to 2006, the incidence of noncardia gastric cancer declined among all race and age groups except for whites aged 25–39 years [6]. While the incidence of gastric cancer has decreased worldwide in recent decades, the incidence of signet-ring cell carcinoma (SRCC) has remained unchanged or even risen in certain parts of the globe [7].

W. F. Barra (✉) · S. Demachki · G. Ishak · P. P. de Assumpção
Núcleo de Pesquisas em Oncologia, Hospital Universitário João de Barros Barreto, Universidade Federal do Pará, Guamá, Belém, Pará, Brazil

© Springer International Publishing AG, part of Springer Nature 2018
T. B. de Castria, R. S. C. Guindalini (eds.), *Diffuse Gastric Cancer*,
https://doi.org/10.1007/978-3-319-95234-5_2

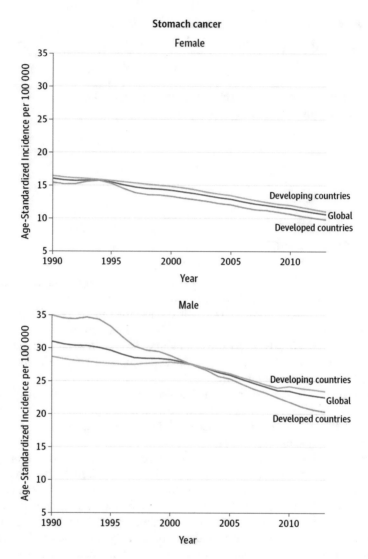

Fig. 2.1 Trends in age-standardized incidence rates for stomach cancer, 1990–2013. (Source: Global Burden of Disease Cancer Collaboration [1])

Age-standardized incidence rates (ASIRs) per 100,000 and age-standardized death rates (ASDRs) per 100,000 for both sexes in 2013 were higher in developing compared to developed countries for stomach cancer (ASIR: 17 vs. 14; ASDR: 15 vs. 11) [7]. Analysis of mortality rates from 1980 to 2005 showed a slower decline in Latin America compared to developed countries (USA, Japan, and Australia) [5].

Diffuse-Type Gastric Carcinoma

The majority of gastric cancers are adenocarcinomas that were classically grouped in the intestinal and diffuse types by the histoclinical Laurén classification in 1965 [8]. Gastric carcinomas represent a biologically and genetically heterogeneous group of tumors with multifactorial etiologies, both environmental and genetic. They are characterized by broad morphological heterogeneity with respect to patterns of architecture and growth, cell differentiation, histogenesis, and molecular pathogenesis.

The World Health Organization (WHO) has categorized gastric cancer into five major histologic types: tubular, papillary, mucinous, poorly cohesive carcinomas (with or without signet ring cell), and mixed. Poorly cohesive carcinoma refers to the diffuse type [9].

Recently, The Cancer Genome Atlas (TCGA) Research Network proposed a molecular gastric cancer classification system that includes four subtypes: Epstein–Barr virus (EBV) positive, microsatellite-unstable, genomically stable, and chromosomal instability (CIN) tumors [10].

The third group, named genomically stable (20% of cases), lacked extensive somatic copy number aberrations, and biopsies often presented a diffuse-type histology. This subtype frequently presented alterations in genes involved in cell adhesion, such as *RHOA* (15%), *CDH1* (26%), and *CLDN18/ARHGAP* (15%). Moreover, these tumors also exhibited elevated expression of cell adhesion and angiogenesis-related pathways [10].

Nevertheless, although the WHO and TCGA classifications brought considerable contributions to the field, Laurén classification is still extensively used in clinical practice.

Compared to intestinal gastric adenocarcinoma, patients with diffuse gastric carcinoma are significantly younger at diagnosis and do not have sex predominance. Patients with diffuse gastric cancer have more advanced and less differentiated tumors, as well as greater invasion depth and lymphovascular invasion [11]. The incidence of intestinal adenocarcinoma decreased faster than that of diffuse carcinoma between 1990 and 2009 in Iceland (0.92/100,000 vs. 0.12/100,000). Median survival rates of diffuse carcinoma were significantly lower than those of intestinal adenocarcinomas [11].

Evaluation of incidence or histologic types among resettlers from the former Soviet Union and the general population in Germany showed that the ASIR of intestinal gastric cancer decreased over time, whereas the ASIR of diffuse gastric cancer remained unchanged [12].

Risk Factors

Environmental Factors

Helicobacter pylori

Helicobacter pylory is a Gram-negative bacterium that colonizes the gastric mucosa. In 1994, the International Agency for Research on Cancer (IARC) categorized *H. pylori* as a Group 1 carcinogen for gastric cancer [13]. *H. pylory* infection is a risk factor for both intestinal and diffuse gastric cancer types [14]. However, in contrast to intestinal-type gastric cancers, diffuse-type gastric cancers have no clearly defined precancerous lesion [15].

Ford et al. (2016) found limited and moderate-quality evidence that searching for and eradicating *H. pylori* reduces the incidence of gastric cancer in healthy asymptomatic infected Asian individuals [16].

There is a risk of developing gastric cancer of both the intestinal and diffuse types even after the eradication of *H. pylori* infection and cessation of gastric inflammation. One survey showed that during follow-up, gastric cancer developed in 28 of 1674 patients up to as much as 13.7 years following the cure of *H. pylori* infection. The risk of developing gastric cancer was 0.30% per year. Histologically, 16 gastric cancers were of the intestinal type and 12 the diffuse type; the risk of each cancer type was 0.17% and 0.13% per year, respectively [17].

Smoking

Smoking causes stomach cancers. Multiple studies in regions with high levels of stomach cancer have shown a small, but significant, increased risk for stomach cancer among smokers [18].

Dietary Habits and Nitroso Compounds

N-nitroso compounds (compounds containing an NO group) are recognized as important dietary carcinogens. N-nitroso compounds are generated following the ingestion of nitrates. Dietary nitrate intake is determined by the type of vegetable consumed, the levels of nitrate in the vegetables (including the nitrate content of fertilizer), the amount of vegetables consumed, and the level of nitrate in the water supply. Diets with high exposure to N-nitroso compounds such as processed meat, smoked and cured fish, and beer have been associated with an increased risk of gastric carcinoma [19]. The IARC reviewed the evidence supporting the linkage between a high intake of processed meat and a variety of cancer sites and concluded that there was a positive association between the consumption of processed meat and stomach cancer [20].

The consumption of total fruit and white vegetables was inversely associated with gastric cancer risk [21]. The protection afforded by vegetables and fruits is most likely related to the presence of dietary nitrosation inhibitors, including vitamin C, which reduce the formation of carcinogenic N-nitroso compounds inside the stomach [22].

Dietary fiber may reduce the risk of gastric cancer, and the association was similar for diffuse-type gastric cancer (OR 0.62, 95% CI 0.42–0.92) and intestinal-type gastric cancer (OR 0.63, 95% CI 0.45–0.89) [23].

Positive associations exist between salt and high-salt foods and gastric cancer risk [21]. The declining incidence of gastric cancer worldwide in recent decades has been attributed in part to the spread of refrigeration [24]. Furthermore, a strong effect of alcohol consumption, particularly beer and liquor but not wine, on gastric cancer risk was observed compared with nondrinkers [21].

Obesity

A meta-analysis showed that excess body weight (body mass index ≥ 25 kg/m^2) was associated with an increased risk of gastric cancer (OR = 1.22, 95% CI = 1.06–1.41) [25]. Specifically, a stratified analysis showed that excess body weight was associated with an increased risk of cardia gastric cancer (OR = 1.55, 95% CI = 1.31–1.84) and gastric cancer among non-Asians (OR = 1.24, 95% CI = 1.14–1.36) [25].

Epstein–Barr Virus

EBV-associated gastric carcinoma is one of the four subtypes of gastric carcinoma, as defined by the novel classification recently proposed by TCGA [8]. It has been estimated that 10% of gastric cancers worldwide are associated with EBV [26].

EBV-associated gastric cancers have male predominance, preferential proximal location, lymphocytic infiltration, less advanced pathologic stage, a diffuse type of histology in most series, and better prognosis [27, 28].

Host Factors

Blood Group

An increased risk of gastric cancer among individuals with blood group A has been identified (incidence ratio = 1.20, 95% CI:1.02–1.42) [29].

CDH1 Gene

Germline pathogenic variants of the *CDH1* gene, which encodes E-cadherin, constitute the genetic causal event of hereditary diffuse gastric cancer (HDGC) [30]. There is evidence that not only germline mutations but also epigenetic changes (e.g., gene promoter hypermethylation) in *CDH1* are associated with the development of gastric cancer, particularly of the diffuse type [31].

HDGC is an inherited form of diffuse-type gastric cancer determined by germline truncating mutations in the *CDH1* gene. Individuals with HDGC face a lifetime cumulative risk of gastric cancer of 70% in men and 56% in women [32].

A model of early development of diffuse gastric cancer in *CDH1* mutation carriers has been proposed, encompassing precursor (intraepithelial) lesions (in situ carcinoma and pagetoid spread of signet ring cells), early intramucosal carcinoma, and advanced cancer [33].

Differences Between Intestinal and Diffuse Subtypes

During data review of the epidemiology of gastric cancer, a range of classic information appears almost constantly: the worldwide incidence varies widely, with developed Western countries tending to have lower incidence; Asian countries have the highest incidence in the world; and, more importantly, gastric cancer incidence and mortality are decreasing due to the reduction of cases of the intestinal subtype [1].

The decrease in the intestinal subtype is usually explained using historical arguments: (a) improvements in food conservation as a consequence of the widespread availability of refrigerators and reduced use of salted food and (b) a decrease in *H. pylori* infection rates caused by improved sanitary conditions and widespread use of antibiotics [21, 24].

These explanations are widely accepted by the scientific community and seem to account for the reduction of intestinal-type incidence and the stable incidence of the diffuse type, which is attributed less to environmental factors and more to genetic factors [30, 31].

Nevertheless, infection with *H. pylori*, recognized by WHO as the strongest known risk factor for gastric cancer, is associated with the development not only of the intestinal type but also of diffuse-type adenocarcinomas [13]. At the same time, some attempts to prove the impact of changes in dietary habits that modify diffuse-type gastric cancer incidence fail to demonstrate significant evidence. In addition, sequential histopathological changes related to the development of diffuse-type gastric cancer remain poorly defined [15].

Taking into consideration that the prevalence of *H. pylori* has been declining in highly industrialized countries of the Western world [34] due to urbanization, sanitation, access to clean water, and improved socioeconomic status, the obvious expected consequence should be a reduction in both the intestinal and diffuse types of gastric cancer.

Based on these data, it is recognized that the reduction in the incidence of gastric cancer is predominantly due to the intestinal subtype. Some differences between the two subtypes is still under investigation, and these differences will be discussed in the following sections.

Age of Occurrence

It is widely known that the diffuse-type gastric cancer seems to occur earlier than the intestinal type [11]. Since it takes many years from *H. pylori* infection to gastric cancer onset, the required time for diffuse-type carcinogenesis should be shorter than that for the occurrence of the intestinal type (a "genetic factor"), and treatment of *H. pylori*, usually prescribed to adult patients, might be irrelevant to diffuse-type tumors, since the necessary molecular steps were already achieved before bacteria eradication. However, the incidence of infection in children has been shown to significantly decrease [34], so the load of the diffuse type could be influenced by this reduction.

Location of Tumors

Intestinal-type gastric cancers are more frequent in the distal stomach, while the diffuse type predominates in proximal regions [11]. Distal tumors incidence decreased and this contributed to reduction of intestinal type cancers, but since distal tumors are not exclusively from the intestinal type, at least a modest decrease in diffuse tumors should be expected.

H. pylori *Infection*

H. pylori infection predominates in the antrum (distal stomach), so a reduction in *H. pylori* infection could explain the reduction of cancer in this part of the stomach. Nevertheless, the carcinogenic pathway attributed to this bacterium is based on corpus infection leading to atrophy, reduced acid secretion, increasing pH, and the subsequent events of carcinogenesis [35].

This mechanism of corpus atrophy, eventually followed by metaplasia, dysplasia, and cancer, as proposed by Correa [35], is thought to partially explain the role of *H. pylori* infection in intestinal-type cancers, but many gaps remain to be filled in our knowledge of diffuse-type carcinogenesis related to *H. pylori* infection.

Reducing microenvironmental acidity is recognized as an important factor favoring gastric carcinogenesis and can be a consequence of both secondary to infection atrophy and medical inhibition of acidity, as largely practiced around the world [36].

The role of reduced acidity via medical therapy in gastric cancer risk remains unproved since pH modification, without additional carcinogenic events, appears to be insufficient to cause cancer [37]. Linking these data to massive *H. pylori* treatment and abusive utilization of proton pump inhibition, a remarkable consequence is a drastic modification in the gastric microenvironment, including the microbiome, which could play a role in the epidemiology of diffuse gastric cancer.

Stomach Microbiome

Before the discovery in 1983 of the occurrence and understanding of the details of *H. pylori* infection pathology, the stomach was thought to be sterile. In 2015, mainly due to new-generation sequencing technologies, a wide variety of microorganisms were discovered to be present in the human stomach; collectively the microorganisms have come to be known as the human gastric microbiota. Increasing evidence supports the hypothesis that, although *H. pylori* may be the most relevant, it is not the only local bacterial culprit leading to gastric diseases [38]. The importance of the gastric microbiome on cancer incidence and even on benign diseases is still under investigation.

Interfering with the Diffuse-Type Gastric Cancer Burden

Many attempts to control the cancer burden have been proposed. For gastric cancer, the treatment of *H. pylori* infection, avoiding salted food, and monitoring patients at risk (relatives of gastric cancer patients, patients with intestinal metaplasia and hereditary cancer syndromes) are the most common measures. Except for HDGC syndrome related to *CDH1* mutations, in which cases prophylactic gastrectomy is recommended, none of the preventive strategies seem to work on diffuse-type tumors since the incidence of these tumors has remained stable [39, 40].

The expected reduction of diffuse-type incidence due to *H. pylori* infection control did not occur, as discussed earlier. Changes in alimentary habits also failed to have an effect, and there are no preneoplastic lesions for diffuse-type cancers, as is the case for metaplasia for the intestinal type.

Diffuse gastric cancer has distinct characteristics of the intestinal subtype. Its incidence remains relatively stable. Further investigation is necessary to elucidate the carcinogenesis and the environmental risk factors that contribute to its development.

References

1. Global Burden of Disease Cancer Collaboration. The global burden of cancer 2013. JAMA Oncol. 2015;1(4):505–27.
2. Parkin DM. Epidemiology of cancer: global patterns and trends. Toxicol Lett. 1998;102–103:227–34.
3. Corso G, et al. History, pathogenesis, and management of familial gastric cancer: original study of John XXIII's family. Biomed Res Int. 2013;2013, 385132
4. Nagini S. Carcinoma of the stomach: a review of epidemiology, pathogenesis, molecular genetics and chemoprevention. World J Gastrointest Oncol. 2012;4(7):156–69.
5. Bertuccio P, et al. Recent patterns in gastric cancer: a global overview. Int J Cancer. 2009;125(3):666.
6. Anderson WF, et al. Age-specific trends in incidence of noncardia gastric cancer in US adults. JAMA. 2010;303(17):1723.
7. Pernot S, Voron T, Perkins G, et al. Signet-ring cell carcinoma of the stomach: Impact on prognosis and specific therapeutic challenge. World J Gastroenterol. 2015;21(40):11428–38.
8. Laurén P. The two histological main types of gastric carcinoma: diffuse and so-called intestinal-type carcinoma. An attempt at a histo-clinical classification. Acta Pathol Microbiol Scand. 1965;64:31–49.
9. Lauwers GY, Carneiro F, Graham DY, et al. Gastric carcinoma. In: Bosman FT, Carneiro F, Hruban RH, Theise ND, editors. WHO classification of tumours of the digestive system. 4th ed. Lyon: IARC; 2010. p. 48–58.
10. The Cancer Genome Atlas Research Network. Comprehensive molecular characterization of gastric adenocarcinoma. Nature. 2014;513:202–9.
11. Chen YC, Fang WL, Wang RF, et al. Clinicopathological variation of Lauren classification in gastric cancer. Pathol Oncol Res. 2016;22(1):197–202.
12. Jaehn P, Holleczek B, Becher H, Winkler V. Histologic types of gastric cancer among migrants from the former Soviet Union and the general population in Germany: what kind of prevention do we need? Eur J Gastroenterol Hepatol. 2016;28(8):863–70.
13. International Agency for Research on Cancer. Schistosomes, liver flukes and Helicobacter pylori. IARC Monogr Eval Carcinog Risk Hum. 1994;61:1–241.
14. Uemura N, Okamoto S, Yamamoto S, et al. Helicobacter pylori infection and the development of gastric cancer. N Engl J Med. 2001;345(11):784–9.
15. Carneiro F, Charlton A, Huntsman DG. Hereditary diffuse gastric cancer. In: Bosman FT, Carneiro F, Hruban RH, Theise ND, editors. WHO classification of tumours of the digestive system. 4th ed. Lyon: IARC; 2010. p. 59–63.
16. Ford AC, Forman D, Hunt R, Yuan Y, Moayyedi P. Helicobacter pylori eradication for the prevention of gastric neoplasia. Cochrane Database Syst Rev. 2015;(7):CD005583.
17. Take S, Mizuno M, Ishiki K, et al. The long-term risk of gastric cancer after the successful eradication of Helicobacter pylori. J Gastroenterol. 2011;46(3):318–24.
18. Sasco AJ, Secretan MB, Straif K. Tobacco smoking and cancer: a brief review of recent epidemiological evidence. Lung Cancer. 2004;45(Suppl 2):S3–9.
19. González CA, Jakszyn P, Pera G, et al. Meat intake and risk of stomach and esophageal adenocarcinoma within the European Prospective Investigation Into Cancer and Nutrition (EPIC). J Natl Cancer Inst. 2006;98:345.
20. Bouvard V, Loomis D, Guyton KZ, et al. Carcinogenicity of consumption of red and processed meat. Lancet Oncol. 2015;16(16):1599–600.
21. Fang X, Wei J, He X, et al. Landscape of dietary factors associated with risk of gastric cancer: a systematic review and dose-response meta-analysis of prospective cohort studies. Eur J Cancer. 2015;51(18):2820–32.
22. Hoang BV, Lee J, Choi IJ, et al. Effect of dietary vitamin C on gastric cancer risk in the Korean population. World J Gastroenterol. 2016;22(27):6257–67.

23. Zhang Z, Xu G, Ma M, Yang J, Liu X. Dietary fiber intake reduces risk for gastric cancer: a meta-analysis. Gastroenterology. 2013;145(1):113.
24. Park B, Shin A, Park SK, et al. Ecological study for refrigerator use, salt, vegetable, and fruit intakes, and gastric cancer. Cancer Causes Control. 2011;22:1497.
25. Yang P, Zhou Y, Chen B, et al. Overweight, obesity and gastric cancer risk: results from a meta-analysis of cohort studies. Eur J Cancer. 2009;45(16):2867–73.
26. Takada K. Epstein-Barr virus and gastric carcinoma. Mol Pathol. 2000;53(5):255.
27. Kusano M, Toyota M, Suzuki H, et al. Genetic, epigenetic, and clinicopathologic features of gastric carcinomas with the CpG island methylator phenotype and an association with Epstein-Barr virus. Cancer. 2006;106(7):1467–79.
28. Lee JH, Kim SH, Han SH, et al. Clinicopathological and molecular characteristics of Epstein-Barr virus-associated gastric carcinoma: a meta-analysis. J Gastroenterol Hepatol. 2009;24(3):354–65.
29. Edgren G, Hialgrim H, Rostgaard K, et al. Risk of gastric cancer and peptic ulcers in relation to ABO blood type: a cohort study. Am J Epidemiol. 2010;172(11):1280–5.
30. Guilford P, Hopkins J, Harraway J, et al. E-cadherin germline mutations in familial gastric cancer. Nature. 1998;392:402–5.
31. Rashid H, Alam K, Afroze D, et al. Hypermethylation status of E-cadherin gene in gastric cancer patients in a high incidence area. Asian Pac J Cancer Prev. 2016;17(6):2757–60.
32. van der Post RS, Vogelaar IP, Carneiro F, et al. Hereditary diffuse gastric cancer: updated clinical guidelines with an emphasis on germline CDH1 mutation carriers. J Med Genet. 2015;52(6):361–74.
33. Carneiro F, Huntsman DG, Smyrk TC, et al. Model of the early development of diffuse gastric cancer in E-cadherin mutation carriers and its implications for patient screening. J Pathol. 2004;203:681–7.
34. McDonald AM, Sarfati D, Baker MG, et al. Trends in Helicobacter pylori infection among Māori, Pacific, and European birth cohorts in New Zealand. Helicobacter. 2015;20(2):139–45.
35. Correa P. Human gastric carcinogenesis: a multistep and multifactorial process – first American Cancer Society Award Lecture on Cancer Epidemiology and Prevention. Cancer Res. 1992;52:6735–40.
36. Haastrup P, Paulsen MS, Zwisler JE, et al. Rapidly increasing prescribing of proton pump inhibitors in primary care despite interventions: a nationwide observational study. Eur J Gen Pract. 2014;20(4):290–3.
37. Attwood SE, Ell C, Galmiche JP, et al. Long-term safety of proton pump inhibitor therapy assessed under controlled, randomised clinical trial conditions: data from the SOPRAN and LOTUS studies. Aliment Pharmacol Ther. 2015;41(11):1162–74.
38. Ianiro G, Molina-Infante J, Gasbarrini A. Gastric microbiota. Helicobacter. 2015;20(Suppl 1):68–71.
39. Henson DE, Dittus C, Younes M, Nguyen H, Albores-Saavedra JA. Differential trends in the intestinal and diffuse types of gastric carcinoma in the United States, 1973–2000: increase in the signet ring cell type. Arch Pathol Lab Med. 2004;128:765–70.
40. Wu H, Rusiecki JA, Zhu K, Potter J, Devesa SS. Stomach carcinoma incidence patterns in the United States by histologic type and anatomic site. Cancer Epidemiol Biomarkers Prev. 2009;18(7):1945–52.

Chapter 3
The Role of Endoscopy

Bruno Frederico Medrado and Bruno da Costa Martins

Preneoplastic Changes

In contrast to intestinal-type cancers, diffuse carcinomas do not have a clearly defined precancerous lesion, even those that are associated with *H. pylori* infection. Histologically, among the diffuse types, signet-ring cell carcinoma (SRCC) is dominant (60%) [15]. Commonly, SRCC of the stomach is thought to arise in the mucosa without metaplastic change and is typically confined to the glandular neck region in the original proliferation zone [16]. It is considered, therefore, that early-stage SRCC can be present beneath a flat, intact mucosal surface epithelium and may be very difficult to identify by endoscopy due to its slightly whitish discoloration.

A representative form of *H. pylori*-negative diffuse gastric cancer, hereditary diffuse gastric cancer (HDGC) cases in early stages, when submitted to histologic analysis, has led to a progression model for the disease [2]. In gastrectomy specimens from members of HDGC families, isolated neoplastic SRCC may be seen at the base of glands, representing an "in situ" carcinoma. Neoplastic cells extend within the epithelium in a "pagetoid" fashion and then invade the stroma in multiple foci [3]. These lesions are thought to represent preinvasive lesions.

B. F. Medrado (✉)
Endoscopy section of Hospital da Clínicas, Faculdade de Medicina da Universidade Federal da Bahia, Salvador, BA, Brazil

B. da Costa Martins
Faculdade de Medicina da Universidade de São Paulo/Instituto do Câncer do Estado de São Paulo, São Paulo, SP, Brazil

© Springer International Publishing AG, part of Springer Nature 2018
T. B. de Castria, R. S. C. Guindalini (eds.), *Diffuse Gastric Cancer*,
https://doi.org/10.1007/978-3-319-95234-5_3

Diagnosis

Detecting an early gastric cancer is a real challenge for the endoscopist. Diffuse early gastric cancer is even harder to diagnosis since mucosal alteration may be subtle. A careful and detailed examination, rinsing out any bubbles and mucous, is essential for spotting an early lesion. Japanese experience underscores the systematic inspection of the stomach, with extensive photodocumentation (>24 images). The location of the tumor in the stomach (cardia, fundus, body, antrum, and pylorus) and its relation to the esophagogastric junction (EGJ) for proximal tumors should be carefully recorded to assist with treatment planning and follow-up examinations [1].

What follow are the characteristics of suspicious-appearing gastric lesions that can be found endoscopically:

- Protrusion
- Redness
- Depression
- Erosion
- Convergence of folds
- Scar
- Loss of vascular pattern
- Bleeding

It is also important to be aware of the following characteristics in order to perform an adequate description of lesions:

- Size and number
- Location (cardia, fundus, body, antrum, pylorus, EGJ)
- Extension (esophagus and duodenum)
- Macroscopic types/endoscopic classifications

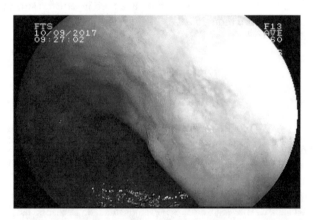

Depressed lesion seen in white light endoscopy.

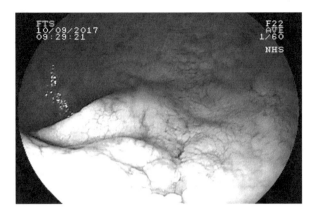

Indigo carmine chromoscopy.

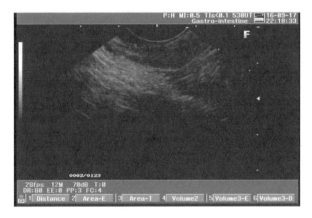

Endosonography showing the involvement of the mucosa, submucosa, and muscular layers.

Chromoendoscopy (CE) involves the topical application of stains or pigments to improve tissue localization, characterization, or diagnosis during endoscopy. Use of methylene blue CE, particularly with magnification, improves identification of gastric lesions. CE with other dyes, such as indigo carmine, acetic acid, and hematoxylin, has also been shown to accurately differentiate between normal gastric mucosa and dysplastic or malignant gastric lesions [17–19].

A meta-analysis of 7 prospective studies, comprising a total of 429 patients and 465 lesions, showed that CE improves the detection of early gastric cancer ($p < 0.01$) and preneoplastic gastric lesions ($p < 0.01$) compared with standard white light examination [20]

In particular, the diagnosis of early diffuse gastric cancer is hampered by the fact that the tumor cells begin infiltrating the mucosa while preserving a normal surface epithelium, and rarely are any visible lesions spotted endoscopically. To overcome this obstacle, a variety of different endoscopic surveillance protocols have been studied in individuals with *CDH1* mutations [21, 22]. Some of these studies demonstrated that CE might increase diagnostic accuracy, and thus the researchers suggested that endoscopy may have a role in guiding the timing of total gastrectomy. However, even in these promising studies, endoscopic surveillance yielded false-negative results in a significant proportion of patients [23].

Endoscopic Classifications

Borrmann classification has been used since 1926 to categorize the macroscopic gross appearance of gastric tumors. This system contemplates only advanced gastric tumors, which are divided into four types:

Type 1: polyploid carcinomas, usually attached on a wide base
Type 2: ulcerated carcinomas with sharply demarcated and raised margins
Type 3: ulcerated, infiltrating carcinomas without definite limits
Type 4: nonulcerated, diffusely infiltrating carcinomas (*linitis plastica*)

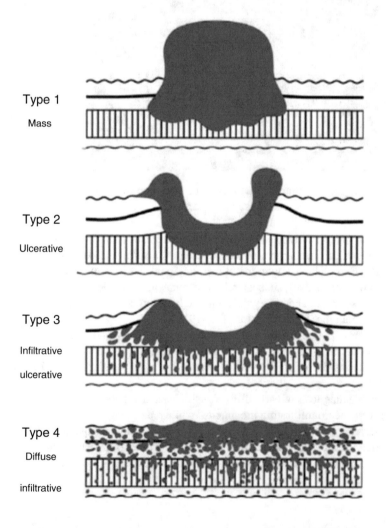

Type 1
Mass

Type 2
Ulcerative

Type 3
Infiltrative
ulcerative

Type 4
Diffuse
infiltrative

Type 0 (superficial)	Typical of T1 tumors.
Type 1 (mass)	Polypoid tumors, sharply demarcated from the surrounding mucosa.
Type 2 (ulcerative)	Ulcerated tumors with raised margins surrounded by a thickened gastric wall with clear margins.
Type 3 (infiltrative ulcerative)	Ulcerated tumors with raised margins, surrounded by a thickened gastric wall without clear margins.
Type 4 (diffuse infiltrative)	Tumors without marked ulceration or raised margins, the gastric wall is thickened and indurated and the margin is unclear.
Type 5 (unclassifiable)	Tumors that cannot be classified into any of the above types.

For early gastric cancers, the Japanese classification, as standardized by the Japanese Gastric Cancer Association (JGCA), is more commonly applied:

- Type I lesions are polypoid or protuberant and are subcategorized as follows:

  - Ip – pedunculated
  - Ips/sp – subpedunculated
  - Is – sessile

- Type II lesions are flat and are further subcategorized as follows:

  - IIa – superficial elevated
  - IIb – flat
  - IIc – flat depressed
  - IIc + IIa lesions – elevated area within a depressed lesion
  - IIa + IIc lesions – depressed area within an elevated lesion

- Type III lesions are ulcerated

A newer classification system for superficial lesions was proposed in 2002, at the workshop of Paris, with the participation of occidental and oriental endoscopists, surgeons, and pathologists. The Paris classification is very similar to the Japanese classification. Superficial lesions (type 0) are classified as polypoid, nonpolypoid, or excavated:

- Type 0-I lesions are polypoid and subcategorized as follows:

  – Type 0-Ip – protruded, pedunculated
  – Type 0-Is – protruded, sessile

- Type 0-II lesions are nonpolypoid and subcategorized as follows:

  – Type 0-IIa – slightly elevated
  – Type 0-IIb – flat
  – Type 0-IIc – slightly depressed

- Type 0-III lesions are excavated

  Mixed types (e.g., 0-IIa + IIc) are classified similarly to the Japanese system.

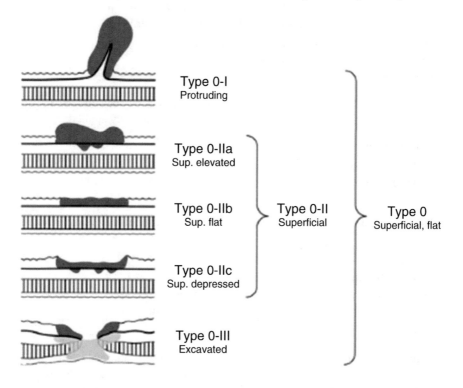

Biopsy

Type 0-I (protruding)[a]	Polypoid tumors.
Type 0-II (superficial)[a]	Tumors with or without minimal elevation or depression relative to the surrounding mucosa.
Type 0-IIa (superficial elevated)[a]	Slightly elevated tumors.
Type 0-IIb (superficial flat)	Tumors without elevation or depression.
Type 0-IIc (superficial depressed)	Slightly depressed tumors.
Type 0-III (excavated)	Tumors with deep depression.

[a] Tumors with less than 3 mm elevation are usually classified as 0-IIa, with more elevated tumors being classified as 0-I

A single biopsy has a 70% sensitivity for diagnosing an existing gastric cancer, while performing seven biopsies from the ulcer margin and base increases the sensitivity to greater than 98% [4]. Multiple (six to eight) biopsies using standard size endoscopy forceps should be performed to provide adequate sized material for histologic interpretation, especially in the setting of an ulcerated lesion. Larger forceps may improve the yield [1]. It is important to point out that if endoscopic resection is being considered, the number of biopsies should be reduced as much as possible (one to three fragments); otherwise the inflammatory response and tissue scarring would difficult the endoscopic approach.

The diagnosis of a particularly aggressive form of diffuse-type gastric cancer, so-called linitis plastica, can be difficult endoscopically. Because these tumors tend to infiltrate the submucosa and muscularis propria, superficial mucosal biopsies may be falsely negative [5]. Poor distensibility of the stomach or the classic appearance on barium swallow (described as a leather flask in appearance) may suggest the presence of this disease.

Endoscopic Ultrasonography Staging

Endoscopic ultrasound (EUS) performed prior to any treatment is important in the initial clinical staging of gastric cancer. Careful attention to ultrasound images provides evidence of depth of tumor invasion (T-category), presence of abnormal or enlarged lymph nodes likely to harbor cancer (N-assessment), and occasionally signs of distant spread, such as lesions in surrounding organs (M-category) or the presence of ascites. This is especially important in patients being considered for endoscopic mucosal resection (EMR) or endoscopic submucosal dissection (ESD) [1].

Endoscopic ultrasound (EUS) accuracy for locoregional staging was recently calculated in a meta-analysis conducted by Mocellin et al., who found the EUS diagnostic accuracy to be clinically useful, mainly to differentiate T1-2 from T3-4 lesions (sensitivity: 86%, specificity: 91%); however, the researchers warned that for T1a/T1b differentiation and node invasion determination, a certain heterogeneity remained to be elucidated for defining the exact role of EUS in the staging of early and advanced gastric cancer [10].

In comparative studies of preoperative staging, EUS generally provides a more accurate prediction of T stage than does computed tomography (CT) [11, 12], although newer CT techniques (such as three-dimensional multidetector row CT) and magnetic resonance imaging may achieve similar results in terms of diagnostic accuracy in T staging [13]

Mainly, EUS is of value for patients with early gastric cancer because accurate assessment of submucosal invasion is essential before considering EMR. Neoadjuvant chemotherapy or chemoradiotherapy may be recommended for patients with a primary tumor that is considered to invade the muscularis propria (T2 or higher) or with a high suspicion of nodal involvement in pretreatment staging studies.

In light of these considerations, EUS is now recommended for pretreatment evaluation of gastric cancer in patients who have no evidence of metastatic (M1) disease in guidelines from the National Comprehensive Cancer Network [1].

Treatment

Correctly identifying disease limited to the mucosa or submucosa (T1 tumors) is key to selecting patients who are suitable for endoscopic treatment. There are usually two options of management: EMR and ESD.

Early Gastric Cancer

The presence of lymph node metastases is considered one of the most significant prognostic factors for overall and disease-free survival in patients with gastric cancer. Therefore, it is essential to highlight the potential lymph node involvement with appropriate surgery and consequently with extended lymphadenectomy but also to propose postoperative chemotherapy when indicated.

In Europe and the USA, the EORTC St. Gallen International Expert Consensus defines the indications for endoscopic resections of early gastric cancer, largely following JGCA guidelines, except for gastric cancers with diffuse histology for which surgery is considered obligatory [6]. Thus, it is not recommended to perform endoscopic resection for early signet-ring cell gastric cancer in Western countries, whatever the depth of invasion in the gastric walls. In Asia, SRCC that is limited to the mucosa, nonulcerated, and less than 2 cm in size can be resected by submucosal endoscopic resection, according to the expanded criteria [7]. Ha et al. [8] supported this indication by demonstrating no lymph node metastasis in 77 patients with early gastric cancer confined to the mucosa, less than 2 cm in size, and with no lymphatic involvement.

Incidence of lymph node metastasis (LNM) in early gastric cancer

Depth of invasion	Tumor size	Ulcerated × not ulcerated	Incidence of LNM	Treatment
Mucosal	<2 cm	Not ulcerated	0%	ESD/surgery
		Ulcerated	2%	Surgery
	2–3 cm	Not ulcerated	1.7%	Surgery
		Ulcerated	2.4%	Surgery
	>3 cm		7.3%	Surgery
Submucosal (sm1)	<3 cm		NC	Surgery
	>3 cm		6.5%	Surgery
Submucosal (sm2)	<3 cm		NC	Surgery
	>3 cm		NC	Surgery

According to Gotoda et al. [9]

Advanced Gastric Cancer

Endoscopic resection is not possible for advanced gastric cancer. Surgical resection is then essential to treat these tumors, combined with an adequate lymphadenectomy, in order to assess the patient's prognosis (proper TNM staging), avoid stage migration, and propose the most appropriate therapeutic strategy. The endoscopist must provide detailed information about tumor location and extension (e.g., distance from cardia, fundus involvement, walls involvement, incisura) for proper surgical planning.

Hereditary Screening

The early gastric cancers that develop in individuals with hereditary inheritance are often multifocal and located beneath an intact mucosal surface [14]. Because of the difficulty in early detection and the poor prognosis of these tumors when locoregionally advanced, patients with evidence of a *CDH1* germline mutation in the context of a family history of HDGC are candidates for prophylactic gastrectomy. However, the timing of this operation may vary according to the preferences and age as well as the physical and psychological fitness of the individual.

For individuals with a *CDH1* mutation in whom gastrectomy is not currently being pursued (e.g., through patient choice or existence of physical or psychological comorbidity), regular endoscopy should be offered (annual). However, patients should be aware that delaying surgery can be hazardous [24].

Due to the tiny *foci* of signet-ring cells, which can only be recognized by microscopy, multiple biopsies are required to maximize the likelihood of diagnosing them [26]. Any endoscopically visible lesions should be biopsied, including pale areas. Additionally, random sampling should be performed; this would involve five biopsies taken from each of the following anatomical zones: prepyloric area, antrum, transitional zone, body, fundus, and cardia. A minimum of 30 biopsies is recommended, as described in the Cambridge protocol [24, 25].

References

1. NCCN Clinical Practice Guidelines in Oncology (NCCN Guidelines®). Gastric cancer, Version 3.2016, NCCN clinical practice guidelines in oncology. J Natl Compr Canc Netw. 2016;14:1286–312.
2. Carneiro F, Huntsman DG, Smyrk TC, Owen DA, Seruca R, Pharoah P, Caldas C, Sobrinho-Simões M. Model of the early development of diffuse gastric cancer in E-cadherin mutation carriers and its implications for patient screening. J Pathol. 2004;203(2):681.
3. Oliveira C, Seruca R, Carneiro F. Genetics, pathology, and clinics of familial gastric cancer. Int J Surg Pathol. 2006;14(1):21.
4. Graham DY, Schwartz JT, Cain GD, Gyorkey F. Prospective evaluation of biopsy number in the diagnosis of esophageal and gastric carcinoma. Gastroenterology. 1982;82(2):228.
5. Karita M, Tada M. Endoscopic and histologic diagnosis of submucosal tumors of the gastrointestinal tract using combined strip biopsy and bite biopsy. Gastrointest Endosc. 1994;40(6):749.
6. Lutz MP, Zalcberg JR, Ducreux M, Ajani JA, Allum W, Aust D, Bang YJ, Cascinu S, Hölscher A, Jankowski J, et al. Highlights of the EORTC St. Gallen international expert consensus on the primary therapy of gastric, gastroesophageal and oesophageal cancer – differential treatment strategies for subtypes of early gastroesophageal cancer. Eur J Cancer. 2012;48:2941–53.
7. Tong JH, Sun Z, Wang ZN, Zhao YH, Huang BJ, Li K, Xu Y, Xu HM. Early gastric cancer with signet-ring cell histologic type: risk factors of lymph node metastasis and indications of endoscopic surgery. Surgery. 2011;149:356–63.
8. Ha TK, An JY, Youn HK, Noh JH, Sohn TS, Kim S. Indication for endoscopic mucosal resection in early signet ring cell gastric cancer. Ann Surg Oncol. 2008;15:508–13.
9. Gotoda T, Yanagisawa A, Sasako M, Ono H, Nakanishi Y, Shimoda T, Kato Y. Incidence of lymph node metastasis from early gastric cancer: estimation with a large number of cases at two large centers. Gastric Cancer. 2000;3:219–25.
10. Mocellin S, Pasquali S. Diagnostic accuracy of endoscopic ultrasonography (EUS) for the preoperative locoregional staging of primary gastric cancer. Cochrane Database Syst Rev. 2015;(2):CD009944.
11. Willis S, Truong S, Gribnitz S, Fass J, Schumpelick V. Endoscopic ultrasonography in the preoperative staging of gastric cancer: accuracy and impact on surgical therapy. Surg Endosc. 2000;14(10):951.
12. Meining A, Dittler HJ, Wolf A, Lorenz R, Schusdziarra V, Siewert JR, Classen M, Höfler H, Rösch T. You get what you expect? A critical appraisal of imaging methodology in endosonographic cancer staging. Gut. 2002;50(5):599.
13. Kwee RM, Kwee TC. Imaging in local staging of gastric cancer: a systematic review. J Clin Oncol. 2007;25(15):2107.
14. Charlton A, Blair V, Shaw D, Parry S, Guilford P, Martin IG. Hereditary diffuse gastric cancer: predominance of multiple foci of signet ring cell carcinoma in distal stomach and transitional zone. Gut. 2004;53(6):814.
15. Matsuo T, Ito M, Takata S, Tanaka S, Yoshihara M, Chayama K. Low prevalence of Helicobacter pylori-negative gastric cancer among Japanese. Helicobacter. 2011;16:415–9.

16. Sugihara H, Hattori T, Fukuda M, Fujita S. Cell proliferation and differentiation in intramucosal and advanced signet ring cell carcinomas of the human stomach. Virchows Arch A Pathol Anat Histopathol. 1987;411:117–27.
17. Tanaka K, Toyoda H, Kadowaki S, et al. Surface pattern classification by enhanced-magnification endoscopy for identifying early gastric cancers. Gastrointest Endosc. 2008;67:430–7. https://doi.org/10.1016/j.gie.2007.10.042.
18. Kono Y, Takenaka R, Kawahara Y, et al. Chromoendoscopy of gastric adenoma using an acetic acid indigocarmine mixture. World J Gastroenterol. 2014;20:5092–7. https://doi.org/10.3748/wjg.v20.i17.5092.
19. Mouzyka S, Fedoseeva A. Chromoendoscopy with hematoxylin in the classification of gastric lesions. Gastric Cancer. 2008;11:15–21 ; discussion 21–2. https://doi.org/10.1007/s10120-007-0445-4.
20. Zhao Z, Yin Z, Wang S, et al. Meta-analysis: the diagnostic efficacy of chromoendoscopy for early gastric cancer and premalignant gastric lesions. J Gastroenterol Hepatol. 2016;31:1539–45. https://doi.org/10.1111/jgh.13313.
21. Shaw D, Blair V, Framp A, et al. Chromoendoscopic surveillance in hereditary diffuse gastric cancer: an alternative to prophylactic gastrectomy? Gut. 2005;54:461–8.
22. Lim YC, di Pietro M, O'Donovan M, et al. Prospective cohort study assessing outcomes of patients from families fulfilling criteria for hereditary diffuse gastric cancer undergoing endoscopic surveillance. Gastrointest Endosc. 2014;80:78–87.
23. Hüneburg R, et al. Chromoendoscopy in combination with random biopsies does not improve detection of gastric cancer foci in CDH1 mutation positive patients. Endosc Int Open. 2016;4(12):E1305–10.
24. Van der Post RS, et al. Hereditary diffuse gastric cancer: updated clinical guidelines with an emphasis on germline CDH1 mutation carriers. J Med Genet. 2015;(52.6):361–74.
25. Fitzgerald RC, Hardwick R, Huntsman D, Carneiro F, Guilford P, Blair V, Chung DC, Norton J, Ragunath K, Van Krieken JH, Dwerryhouse S, Caldas C. International gastric cancer linkage C. Hereditary diffuse gastric cancer: updated consensus guidelines for clinical management and directions for future research. J Med Genet. 2010;47:436–44. https://doi.org/10.1136/jmg.2009.074237.
26. Barber M, Murrell A, Ito Y, Maia AT, Hyland S, Oliveira C, Save V, Carneiro F, Paterson AL, Grehan N, Dwerryhouse S, Lao-Sirieix P, Caldas C, Fitzgerald RC. Mechanisms and sequelae of E-cadherin silencing in hereditary diffuse gastric cancer. J Pathol. 2008;216:295–306. https://doi.org/10.1002/path.2426.

Chapter 4
Pathology and Molecular Biology

Maria Aparecida Azevedo Koike Folgueira,
Marina Candido Visontai Cormedi, Daniela Marques Saccaro,
and Maria Lucia Hirata Katayama

Molecular Biology of Gastric Cancer

The Cancer Genome Atlas (TCGA) (2014), based on dysregulated pathways and candidate driver genes, has divided gastric cancer (GC) cases into four subtypes: Epstein-Barr virus (*EBV*)-infected tumors, microsatellite instability (*MSI*) tumors, genomically stable (*GS*) tumors, and chromosomal instability (*CIN*) tumors. The main characteristics of this classification are described in what follows.

According to the TCGA, around 50% of GC cases may be classified as chromosomally unstable, featuring marked aneuploidy, high somatic copy number alterations (SCNA), including focal amplification of receptor tyrosine kinases, such as ERBB2, EGFR, ERBB3, *FGFR2*, MET, *KRAS*, and *VEGFA*, as well as cell cycle mediators, such as CCNE1, CCND1, and CDK6, most of them amenable to targeted therapies. In addition, DNA hypomethylation and a high frequency of TP53 mutation may also be detected [1]. Another 9% of cases may be classified as positive for EBV, an alteration that may be accompanied by phosphatidylinositol-4,5-bisphosphate 3-kinase catalytic subunit alpha (PIK3CA) mutations, DNA hypermethylation, including cyclin-dependent kinase inhibitor, also known as p16^{INK4A} (*CDKN2A*) silencing. Other alterations are amplifications of Janus kinase 2 (JAK2), CD274 (also known as PD-L1), and programmed cell death 1 ligand 2, also known as PD-L2 (PDCD1LG2), that may be accompanied by mRNA increased expression, indicating implication of immune signaling. Another 20% of GC cases may be classified as microsatellite unstable tumors, showing elevated mutation rates, including mutations of genes encoding targetable oncogenic signaling proteins. In most of these cases, the mismatch repair defect is more likely due to an epigenetic hypermethylation in the MLH1 promoter region. In addition, microsatellite unstable GCs are generally intestinal-type tumors, according to Lauren's classification. Finally,

M. A. A. K. Folgueira (✉) · M. C. V. Cormedi · D. M. Saccaro · M. L. H. Katayama
Faculdade de Medicina FMUSP, Universidade de Sao Paulo, Sao Paulo, SP, BR
e-mail: maria.folgueira@fm.usp.br

© Springer International Publishing AG, part of Springer Nature 2018
T. B. de Castria, R. S. C. Guindalini (eds.), *Diffuse Gastric Cancer*,
https://doi.org/10.1007/978-3-319-95234-5_4

20% of cases may be classified as GS tumors, which are enriched for the diffuse histological variant and for mutations in *CDH1* (E-cadherin) or ras homolog family, member A (*RHOA*), or fusions involving Rho-family GTPase-activating proteins [1–3].

Another extensive molecular analysis was performed by the Asian Cancer Research Group (ACRG). Based on gene expression signatures, this group also identified four GC subtypes; however, they do not totally correspond to TCGA classification. In this analysis, GC samples were separated in microsatellite unstable (*MSI*) or microsatellite stable (MSS) tumors, which were further divided into tumors with epithelial-to-mesenchymal transition (*MSS-EMT*) signature, tumors with functional loss of TP53 (*MSS-TP53⁻*), and tumors with intact TP53 (*MSS-TP53+*). In this analysis, TP53 activation status was evaluated using a two-gene (CDKN1A, also known as p21, and *MDM2*) signature, in which a high score defines tumors with intact TP53 activity and vice versa [1, 2].

Following the ACRG expression signatures, the *MSI* subtype accounts for 22.7% of tumors and is enriched in intestinal tumors. This subtype is associated with a loss of expression of MLH1, elevated DNA methylation signature, and hypermutation, with alterations in genes such as *KRAS*, the PI3K-PTEN-mTOR pathway, ALK, ARID1A, and PIK3CA. Around 15% of the samples may be classified as being of the *MSS-EMT* subtype, which is enriched in diffuse Lauren histology. In MSS-EMT, loss of *CDH1* expression, as well as a lower number of somatic mutations and copy number variations, is more frequently found than in the other subtypes. Another 35.7% of tumors are *MSS-TP53⁻* and present low TP53 activity (low CDKN1A and *MDM2* scores) and a high TP53 mutation rate. The remaining 26.3% of cases are classified as *MSS-TP53+*, which present a lower TP53 mutation rate but a relatively higher prevalence of mutations in APC, ARID1A, *KRAS*, PIK3CA, and SMAD4 than *MSS-TP53⁻*. In addition, in *MSS-TP53+*, EBV infection is more frequently detected [2].

Although a comparison between the TCGA and ACRG classifications shows similarities, it also reveals important differences. Among the similarities is the fact that there is an association between GC samples classified as MSI subtype, using both data sets. In addition, TCGA subtypes GS, EBV⁺, and CIN are enriched in samples classified as MSS/EMT, MSS/TP53⁺, and MSS/TP53⁻, respectively, according to ACRG. However, some differences may be detected when analyzing tumors with Lauren's diffuse histology. In addition, tumors classified as CIN, according to TCGA, may be classified in all four ACRG subtypes. Furthermore, even though EBV⁺ cases were more frequently detected in the MSS/TP53⁺ subtype, they represented only a small proportion of samples (around 15%) from this subtype, suggesting that these correlations were also weak [1, 2].

Although GC studies have been increasing lately, few works have been dedicated solely to diffuse gastric cancer (DGC). According to the TCGA classification, the GS subtype is enriched in tumors with diffuse histology; these represent 73% of samples. However, among all tumor samples analyzed by this group, only 19% were characterized as GS. Considering all DGC included in the TCGA study, around 60% of DGCs were characterized as GS and the remaining 40% were classified in each of the other subgroups, mainly CIN (28%), followed by MSI and EBV (6% each). In the ACRG analysis, the MSS-EMT subtype was enriched in samples with diffuse histology, which represented around 85% of MSS-EMT tumors. However, as reported earlier, only 15% of all the samples analyzed by the ACRG were classified as MSS-EMT. Hence, considering all DGC cases included in the analysis, 27% were classified as MSS-EMT, and the remaining diffuse tumors were characterized as MSS-TP53⁻ (31%), MSS-TP53⁺ (27%), and MSI (15%).

Considering both studies, a higher percentage of tumors with Lauren's diffuse histology was analyzed in the ACRG (45%) than in the TCGA (24%), and in the latter, diffuse tumors seemed less heterogeneous. In addition, *CDH1* and *RHOA* alterations, which correlate to the diffuse tumors and GS subtype (TCGA), were not frequent in the MSS-EMT subtype (ACRG). These differences suggest that the TCGA GS subtype is not equivalent to the ACRG MSS-EMT subtype [1, 2].

In the following paragraphs, we will describe the main characteristics of DGC, sometimes using data obtained for this specific Lauren's histological subtype and sometimes using data generated in GS tumors or MSS-EMT tumors, with the latter two subtypes mainly comprising DGC samples.

Genomic Alterations

Genes located at the same position (*locus*) in homologous chromosomes are known as alleles, and those alleles that are found more frequently in a population are known as wild-type alleles. When an alteration of the nucleotide sequence of the gene occurs, such as a substitution, an insertion, or a deletion, a new, mutant allele appears. These mutations may occur in germline cells, and therefore be hereditary, or they may occur sporadically in somatic cells, and in this case, they are not transmitted to the offspring. If the alteration is a small deletion or insertion, it may change the reading frame of the gene, and it is called a frame shift. This kind of mutation is likely pathogenic, leading to a dysfunctional protein and possibly to a disease. In addition, if a nucleotide substitution happens, it may create a stop codon (nonsense) or change a splicing sequence, which also gives rise to a dysfunctional protein. Otherwise, benign substitutions are silent and do not alter the protein function.

Copy number variations (CNVs) are alterations involving larger stretches of chromosomal DNA. When the alteration increases, decreases, or annihilates the number of copies of a gene (called amplification or deletion), it may lead to an overexpression, underexpression, or total absence of the protein, respectively. A mutation may also change the gene sequence in a chromosome, which is known as a translocation, usually engendering a chimeric protein whose function will be different from that of the original. Translocations may involve the breaking and rebinding of genes in the same chromosome or the exchange of DNA between different chromosomes. Moreover, many gene mutations are of unknown significance.

Let us first review somatic mutations associated with DGC and GS tumors. The genes most frequently mutated in DGC, according to COSMIC (Catalogue of

Table 4.1 Genes most frequently mutated in DGC

Gene	Name	Functional group	Role in carcinogenesis
CDH1	E-cadherin 1	Cell adhesion	Tumor suppressor
RHOA	Ras homolog family member A	Cytoskeleton and cell motility	Unknown (see section on RHOA pathway)
TP53	Tumor protein p53	Genome integrity	Tumor suppressor
ARID1A	AT-rich interaction domain 1A	Chromatin remodeling	Tumor suppressor
PIK3CA	Phosphatidylinositol-4,5-bisphosphate 3-kinase catalytic subunit alpha	Receptor tyrosine kinase pathway	Oncogene
KRAS	Kirsten rat sarcoma viral oncogene homolog	Receptor tyrosine kinase/cell cycle	Oncogene
CTNNB1	Catenin beta 1	Cell adhesion/ Wnt-signaling pathway	Oncogene

Somatic Mutation in Cancer), include *TP53* (39%), *CDH1* (23%), *ARID1A* (20%), *RHOA* (13%), *PIK3CA* (8%), and *SMAD4* (7,5%). Similarly, in GS tumors, somatic mutations are most frequently found in genes such as *CDH1* (cadherin 1), *RHOA*, *ARID1A*, *PIK3CA*, *TP53*, *KRAS*, and *CTNNB1*. Table 4.1 describes the main functions and roles of these genes in carcinogenesis [4]. Other whole-genome (exome) sequencing studies reported similar results [5, 6].

In GS tumors, *CDH1* somatic mutation is relatively frequent (37% of tumors, mainly missense), but generally it is not concomitant with *TP53* mutation [1]. In studies analyzing specifically DGC, the proportion of *CDH1* mutation varies between 23% and 33% and is significantly higher than in other histological and molecular subtypes. The most frequent type of mutation is missense, leading to a dysfunctional protein that impairs cell adhesion [1, 5, 6].

RHOA, involved in actin organization and cell migration, is another frequently mutated gene in GS tumors as well as in DGC. Notably, *RHOA* mutations are found only in DGC, in which its frequency varies between 10% and 25%. The most common alterations are missense, but whether those lead to a gain or loss of function remains unclear. Nevertheless, recent findings indicate that *RHOA* may be a driver mutation in the diffuse histological subtype [1, 5–7]. In addition, dysregulated RHO signaling may also be detected as interchromosomal translocations between Rho-family GTPase-activating proteins, such as *CLDN18* and *ARHGAP26* (GRAF) or *CLDN18-ARHGAP6*. Together, these mutually exclusive alterations may be found in 30% of GS tumors. Another chromosomal translocation described in DGC is *SLC34A2-ROS1*, which affects a gene that codes a receptor tyrosine kinase [1, 8].

Considering SCNA, the most frequently reported in GS tumors are focal amplifications targeting genes such as *VEGFA*, *GATA4*, *MYC*, *FGFR2*, *CD44*, 11q14.1, *KRAS*, 12q13.11, *MDM2*, 15q26.1, and Xq27.3. In addition, focal deletions targeting regions 2q32.1, 3p24.1, 4q25, *PTPRD*, *CDKN2A*, 18q23, Xq21.23, including genes localized at fragile sites such as *FAM190A*, *PDEA4D*, *IMMP2L*, *WWOX*, and *MACROD2*, were also described in GS tumors [1].

Epigenetics

The modification in the DNA sequence of oncogenes and tumor suppressor genes is well known and characterized in cancer. Additionally, chromatin structure and organization have a significant effect on gene expression. The study of heritable changes in gene expression that occur independently of changes in DNA sequence is called epigenetics. In the past decade, the role of epigenetic abnormalities in cancer pathogenesis has been extensively investigated.

The main epigenetic mechanisms include changes in DNA methylation profile, histone modifications, and abnormalities of microRNA expression or binding. In this section, the contribution of these alterations for DGC will be discussed.

DNA Methylation

The process of DNA methylation is the most studied epigenetic modification. It occurs in chromatin sequences rich in CpG dinucleotides, usually clustered in regions called CpG islands. The methylation status of a CpG island is associated with gene-expression variation. When a DNA region loses its methyl group or a methyl is added in a position usually unmethylated, this is called hypomethylation and hypermethylation, respectively. (Sharma et al. 2009). The enzymes responsible for the transfer of methyl groups to the DNA are called DNA methyltransferases (DNMT).

Cancer is known for presenting a conflicting epigenetic profile: global hypomethylation and gene-specific hypermethylation. Global hypomethylation is considered one of cancer's hallmarks and is believed to be associated with the disease by the mechanisms of chromosomal instability, reactivation of transposable elements, and loss of imprinting. Otherwise, hypermethylation of CpG islands in gene promoters is associated with gene silencing and loss of protein expression [9].

According to TGCA, GS and CIN tumors have similar hypermethylation profiles, which are less prominent than EBV and MSI subtypes. Nevertheless, when MSS non-EBV tumors are reclassified according to histological subtype, DGCs present higher rates of CpG island methylation, whereas intestinal tumors show a higher chromosomal instability index and more widespread demethylation of the genome [1, 5].

In DGC, the best characterized gene that undergoes promoter hypermethylation is *CDH1*, which codifies the cell-adhesion protein, epithelial cadherin (E-cadherin) 1. The methylation of *CDH1* promoter is largely found in gastric tumors and can lead to gene silencing and reduced protein expression. This is one of the possible mechanisms involved in the complete inactivation of the *CDH1* gene in hereditary DGC and sporadic DGC [10].

Considering DNA methyltransferases, some aberrant patterns have been described in gastric tumors. Overexpression of DNMT 1, 3A and 3B in stomach neoplastic tissue was reported in some studies, and seems to be associated with clinicopathological features. DNMT3A levels were linked to tumor stage and lymph node metastasis, and higher levels of DNMT3B were related to lymph node metastasis. Although these findings represent an advance in epigenetic knowledge, the cause and consequences of this enzyme's expression is not fully understood. Therefore, the role of the DNMT family is likely extensive in gastric carcinogenesis, but the specific correlation with the diffuse subtype is yet to be investigated [11].

Histone Alterations

Histones are proteins that bind to DNA, providing stability to chromatin. The interaction between histones and DNA determines the accessibility of chromatin to the transcription apparatus. Generally, acetylated histones allow transcription factors to interact with chromatin, to induce DNA transcription, in contrast to methylated histones, which tend to decrease DNA transcription. In GC, methylation of histones, such as H3K27me3 and H3K9me3, are associated with poorer prognosis by inactivating tumor suppressor genes [11]. There is no described pattern of histone modification specific to DGC.

MicroRNA

MicroRNA (miRNA) constitutes another layer of gene-expression regulation. MiRNAs are small noncoding RNA sequences of approximately 22 nucleotides that may interact through base pairing with complementary sequences in the 3′ untranslated region (3′ UTR) of messenger RNAs (mRNAs) to target them for degradation and thereby prevent their translation. More than 1000 individual miRNAs have been identified, and each one can target a great number of different mRNAs. miRNAs can control cell proliferation, differentiation, and survival, among other processes, so changes in miRNA expression patterns may be involved in tumor development [12].

According to the TCGA, some miRNA (miR) such as miR-1, miR-133a-3p, miR-133b, miR-145-3p, miR-143-3p, miR-490-3p, let-7c-5p, miR-125b-2-3p, and miR-99a-5p are relatively more expressed in GS tumors, compared to the other subtypes. However, these same miRNAs are similarly expressed between GS tumors and gastric normal tissue [1].

In another study, the TCGA database was reevaluated to characterize miRNAs expressed in diffuse and intestinal histological subtypes. The miRNAs 100-5p, 195, let-7c-5p, 140, 99a-5p, and 125-b2-3p were correlated with the diffuse subtype, while miRNAs 210, 592, 130b, and 455 were associated with the intestinal subtype [1, 13]. The miRNAs 100-5p, 99a-5p, and 125-b2-3p may be involved in the regulation of hematopoietic stem cells by TGFbeta and Wnt signaling pathways. We have further explored this miRNA data to identify mRNA target candidates using miRWalk 2.0: a comprehensive atlas of predicted and validated miRNA-target interactions [14], followed by Toppgene suite, to perform gene list enrichment analysis and candidate gene prioritization [15]. Potential targets for miR let-7c-5p are genes such as

MAP3K1, *RANBP2*, *EIF2S2*, *CTPS2*, *ZNF341*, and *FNIP1*, and biological processes enriched in these genes are "de novo" CTP biosynthetic process, positive regulation of B-cell apoptotic process, positive regulation of protein complex assembly (*MAP3K1* and *FNIP1*), and regulation of pro-B cell differentiation; the targets for miR 99a-5p/100-5p are mainly *EMR2*, *USP12*, *HSD3B7*, *IMPDH1*, *TNFAIP8L1*, *C20orf194*, *CAND2*, *MYCBP*, *TRIB2*, *FOXJ3*, *RRN3*, *ICMT*, *ZZEF*, *SETD1B*, *KDM6B*, and *ALG13*, and enriched biological processes are the negative regulation of interleukin-T10 biosynthetic process (*TRIB2*), SCF complex assembly (*CAND2*), regulation of interleukin-10 biosynthetic process (*TRIB2*), and C-terminal protein methylation (*ICMT*); the targets for miR 125-b2-3p are *KCNT1*, *KLC1*, *RPL28*, *CCPG1*, *SLC35D2*, *PCMTD2*, and *NSFL1C*, and the biological process enriched are the regulation of Rho guanyl-nucleotide exchange factor activity (*CCPG1*), stress granule disassembly (*KLC1*), regulation of guanyl-nucleotide exchange factor activity (*CCPG1*), pyrimidine nucleotide-sugar transmembrane transport (*SLC35D2*), and organelle disassembly (*KLC1*, *RPL28*).

Gene and Protein Expression

A way to further improve the characterization of GC subtypes has been through differential gene expression analysis, especially through cDNA microarray, where the information coded by all transcribed genes may be considered.

Analysis of the TCGA database, using RNA seq data sets, revealed 40 differentially expressed genes that might classify the groups MSI, CIN, EBV, and GS. Among these genes, 10 were more expressed in GS tumors in relation to CIN, MIS, and EBV: *FLNC*, *HSPB6*, *ACTG2*, *CNN1*, *DES*, *HSPB7*, *LYOD1*, *MYH11*, *SYNPO2*, and *SYNM*. Using ToppGene analysis, biological process enriched in these genes were muscle contraction (*HSPB6*, *ACTG2*, *CNN1*, *DES*, *MYH11*, *SYNM*); regulation of system process (*HSPB6*, *CNN1*, *DES*, *HSPB7*); actin filament-based process (*FLNC*, *CNN1*, *DES*, *MYH11*); and intermediate filament cytoskeleton organization (*SYN*, *DES*). However, the expression of these genes was similar in the comparison between normal tissue and GS tumors. In addition, some genes were differentially abundant only between GS group versus adjacent normal tissue, some more expressed (*SFRP4*, *CLDN3*, *THBS4*, *THBS2*, *CST1*, *BGN*, *FNDC1*, *COL8A1*, *ASPN*) and others less expressed (*GKN1*, *GKN2*, *LIPF*, *PGC*, *TFF2*, *GIF*, *REG3A*, *PGA3*, *PSCA*, *CXCL17*) in GS tumors [1].

In another attempt to better classify the histological subtypes, it was shown that genes overexpressed in diffuse tumors code for proteins involved in extracellular matrix processes. In this work, thrombospondin 4 (THBS4), an important adhesive glycoprotein, was more expressed in diffuse than intestinal subtypes. In addition, using immunohistochemistry, it was shown that THBS4 may be detected specifically in the stromal compartment of diffuse tumors [16].

Further studies used microdissected diffuse-type GC, as compared to their corresponding noncancerous mucosae, to reveal differentially expressed genes that might be involved in carcinogenesis and tumor progression. Genes more expressed in tumor samples included *COL3A1*, *TGFB1*, *SPARC*, *MSLN*, *FLJ20736*, *GW112*, *EST* (*AA430699*), and *EST* (*AA143060*). In addition, comparison of the expression profiles of the diffuse type with those of the intestinal type demonstrated 46 differentially expressed genes. Fourteen genes were more expressed in the diffuse type, including those encoding chaperones (*CCT3* and *TOR1B*) or associated with cell motility and cytoskeleton (*CD81* and *TUBA3*) and glycosylation (*RPN2*, *MGAT1*, and *MPI*). Another 32 genes were more expressed in diffuse-type tumors, such as those involved in signal transduction and transcriptional regulation (*RHBDL*, *SFRS8*, *MLL5*, *LDB3*, and *GFRA2*), nuclear transportation (*KPNB2* and *NUP133*) and cell adhesion (*PSK-1, ITGB5, SRPX* and *IBSP*). In conclusion, this study identified genes that could distinguish different mechanisms underlying gastric carcinogenesis [17].

Proteomic analysis of GS tumors may also add some clues to tumor behavior. Increased protein expression of *CAV1*, *MYH11*, and *RICTOR* and reduced expression of *CTNNB1* (Catenin Beta 1), *CDH1*, and *MTOR* in GS tumors as compared to other subtypes of GC was described. Other proteins that may be less expressed in GS tumors, as compared with MSI-H, EBV e CIN subtypes, were KIT, HSP70, *MYC*, PRKCA, PRKCA pS657, CCND1 (Cyclin D1), EIF4EBP1 pS65, ACVRL1, BCL2, TUBA acetyl Lys40, CoOl6A1, PKC-pan pS660, PEA15, and AKT [1].

Finally, expression of some genes, such as *HER2*, are particularly important due to their clinical relevance. For example, *HER2-neu* overexpression, used to indicate trastuzumab treatment, is detected in only a small percentage of diffuse histology cancers, around 6%, in contrast with 32% of the intestinal histology cases [18].

Pathways

Hierarchical clustering of samples and pathways revealed that the GS subtype exhibited elevated expression of cell-adhesion pathways, including the B1/B3 integrins, syndecan-1-mediated signaling, and angiogenesis-related pathways in contrast to other subtypes (CIN, EBV, MSI), which exhibited elevated expression of mitotic network components such as AURKA/B and E2F, targets of *MYC* activation, FOXM1 and PLK1 signaling, and DNA damage response pathways [1].

Specifically, one molecule involved in the cell-adhesion pathway deserves further attention regarding its mechanism of regulation: E-cadherin.

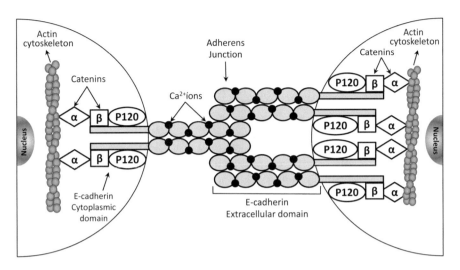

Fig. 4.1 Cell adhesion mediated by E-cadherin. E-cadherin homodimerizes in the presence of calcium ions and binds to other E-cadherin molecules from an adjacent cell through the extracellular domain; p120 catenin and β-catenin interact with the E-cadherin cytoplasmic domain. Subsequently, β-catenin interacts with α-catenin, which then anchors the structure to the actin cytoskeleton

E-Cadherin and Cell Adhesion

E-cadherin is encoded by the *CDH1* gene, which is located on chromosome 16q22.1 and is composed of 16 exons and 15 introns. E-cadherin belongs to the family of cell-adhesion molecules and plays a fundamental role in the maintenance of cell differentiation and the normal architecture of epithelial tissues [19].

E-cadherin is composed of three major structural domains: an extracellular domain, comprising five tandemly repeated domains, EC1–EC5; a single transmembrane domain; and a cytoplasmic domain. The extracellular domain is involved in cell adhesion, through homodimerization with cadherins from adjacent cells, in the presence of calcium ions. The cytoplasmic domain includes the juxtamembrane domain, which interacts with p120-catenin and the catenin-binding domain, which binds beta-catenin and gamma-catenin. In a second step, beta-catenin binds to alfa-catenin, which is anchored to the actin cytoskeleton, establishing the cadherin–catenin complex (Fig. 4.1). The stability of the cadherin–catenin complex and its linkage to actin filaments form the core of the adherens junction, which is vital in the inhibition of individual epithelial cell motility and in providing homeostatic tissue architecture [19].

E-Cadherin and the Wnt/Beta-Catenin Signaling Pathway

Wnt and cadherin pathways are important in the regulation of beta-catenin activity. Extracellular Wnt proteins bind to cell surface receptors of the Frizzled family, promoting beta-catenin translocation from the cytoplasm to the nucleus. In the nucleus, beta-catenin activates transcription factors, such as TCF and LEF, inducing the transcription of target genes involved in cell migration, cell proliferation, and apoptosis [20].

Beta-catenin can be found in the membrane, cytoplasm, or nucleus depending on the status of Wnt signals and the expression and distribution of E-cadherin. In most cases, overexpression of E-cadherin inhibits beta-catenin transcriptional activity. Contrariwise, when Wnt signaling is active or when E-cadherin is phosphorylated by a tyrosine kinase, it releases beta-catenin. The latter then accumulates in the cytoplasm and translocates to the nucleus, where it can then regulate the transcription [19, 21].

E-Cadherin and Epithelial-to-Mesenchymal Transition

There is accumulating evidence that epithelial–mesenchymal transition (EMT) is involved in GC aggressiveness. EMT is a biological process that allows a polarized epithelial cell (adherent cell) to undergo multiple biochemical changes that enable it to assume a mesenchymal cell phenotype, including enhanced migratory capacity, invasiveness, and elevated resistance to apoptosis [22]. When cells undergo EMT, they lose E-cadherin, dissolve cell adhesions, and are prone to invading adjacent tissues and metastasizing. Hence, maintaining adequate E-cadherin levels is an important mechanism to preserve tissue architecture and inhibit the invasion of adjacent tissues [23].

E-Cadherin Expression and Function

CDH1 may be considered a tumor suppressor gene, linked with human cancer susceptibility [24]. Consequently, abrogation of E-cadherin function, through genetic, epigenetic, or posttranslational mechanisms, may be a carcinogenic event. Besides gene mutations, other mechanisms that may be involved in *CDH1* downregulation include promoter methylation or upregulation of transcriptional repressors.

E-cadherin immunoreactivity is often reduced or lost in less differentiated and invasive diffuse carcinomas. E-cadherin aberrant immunoreactions have been observed significantly more frequently in the diffuse-type carcinomas (82.4%) in comparison to the intestinal-type carcinomas (31.6%), emphasizing the strong relation between Lauren's classification of gastric carcinomas and the immunohistochemical expression of the E-cadherin cellular adhesion molecule [25].

Germline and Somatic Mutations in *CDH1* Gene

Sporadic *CDH1* genetic and epigenetic alterations were described earlier in this chapter. In summary, 23–33% of DGCs present *CDH1* mutations, leading to defective cell-adhesion function, and epigenetic silencing of the gene promoter by methylation is very frequently associated with low E-cadherin expression [1, 5, 6, 10]. Hereditary genetic and epigenetic alterations in *CDH1* are discussed elsewhere (Chap. 5).

Transcriptional Regulation of E-Cadherin Expression

Transcriptional control is an essential regulatory mechanism of E-cadherin expression. The characterization of an E-cadherin promoter region revealed several potential proximal regulatory elements: a CCAAT box (−65), a GC-rich region (−30 to −58), and a palindromic element (−70 to −90), composed of adjacent E-boxes, flanked by four inverted nucleotides called Epal. The proximal CCAAT and GC-rich regions, which are recognized by constitutive AP2 and Sp1 transcriptional factors and CAAT-binding proteins, respectively, are required for basal E-cadherin expression [26].

A major breakthrough in understanding the regulation of E-cadherin transcription was the identification of several E-cadherin repressors. These transcriptional repressors, represented by the zinc finger factors Snail and Slug (another member of the Snail family), as well as by class I basic region helix–loop–helix (bHLH) factor E47, specifically bind to the E-boxes and overcome the positive effects of constitutive factors. In addition, another two factors of the zinc finger family, Zeb1 and Zeb2, have also been described as repressors of E-cadherin.

Functional characterization of Snail indicates that it does indeed act as a strong repressor of the E-cadherin promoter. Snail repressor activity apparently requires three E-boxes of the human promoter. Importantly, overexpression of Snail in epithelial cells produces a dramatic EMT and promotes the acquisition of migratory and in vitro invasive behavior [27]. E47 and Slug were also shown to behave as E-cadherin repressors and to induce EMT when overexpressed in epithelial cell lines [26].

Posttranslational Regulation of E-Cadherin Expression

E-cadherin cellular levels may also be regulated through posttranslational modifications, such as phosphorylation, glycosylation, and proteolytic processing. Some important players in this process are p120 catenin and Hakai. Binding of p120 catenin with the cadherin juxtamembrane domain stabilizes and suppresses cadherin endocytosis and promotes the formation of adherens junctions. Removal of p120 from the cadherin complex, via phosphorylation of p120, uncovers an adaptor protein 2 (AP-2) binding motif, as well as a phosphorylation-dependent motif for the recruitment of the E3 ligase Hakai. AP-2 binding promotes clathrin-dependent endocytosis of E-cadherin, which can subsequently be recycled back to the membrane. Otherwise, the endocytosed E-cadherin may be a target of Hakai-induced ubiquitination followed by degradation in the proteasome [28].

RHOA Pathway

RHOA is a member of the RAS superfamily, which is known to be involved in cell proliferation. *RHOA* is a small GTPase, encoded by a gene in chromosome 3, and it is highly conserved in species over the course of evolution. It participates in numerous biological processes by functioning as a molecular switch in signal transduction cascades. Rho proteins promote actin polymerization and regulate cell shape, attachment, and motility. They are also involved with cell cycle progression.

Recently, *RHOA* mutations have been described by whole-genome sequencing in GC studies as being exclusive to DGC or GS and a possible new driver of this subtype of diseases. Most *RHOA* alterations occur in functional domains involved in GTP binding and interaction with effectors designed as hotspots. Whether these mutations promote gain or loss of *RHOA* function is not clear. The evidence of loss of heterozygosity and anoikis escape in cells with mutated *RHOA* indicates loss of function, while growth-promoting effects in cells and bioinformatic analysis showing activation of *RHOA* pathways with mutated gene variants suggests gain of function. These data may indicate that, even though mutant *RHOA* lose their GTP-binding capacity, they may acquire a new oncogenic activity, perhaps by an unidentified signaling pathway [7].

The *RHOA* signaling pathway may also be altered by a recently described chromosomal translocation. CLDN18-ARHGAP26 is a fusion protein recurrently screened in GC samples. ARHGAP26 negatively regulates *RHOA* activity via the GAP domain. Under the influence of CLDN18 promoter, ARHGAP26 inactivates *RHOA*, and as a result, the actin cytoskeleton and cell-to-cell adhesion are affected. Therefore, epithelial tissue is damaged and its cells may not be replaced, promoting gaps that enhance tissue injury and may eventually lead to GC [1].

The nature of interaction between *RHOA* and *CDH1* is of importance for understanding DGC molecular pathology. A missense mutation on the extracellular domain of E-cadherin is believed to be responsible for increased cell motility in a mechanism involving *RHOA* activation. E-cadherin mutants show reduced stability of E-cadherin/EGFR heterodimers. This results in their disruption and EGF activation of homodimers, which leads to *RHOA* activation and increased cell motility. These data give new insights into the understanding of mechanisms linking invasion and E-cadherin mutations in DGC [29].

These new findings place *RHOA* as an important candidate gene target for new therapies in DGC.

Survival According to Molecular Subtypes

The diffuse-type GC, according to Lauren classification and description, is associated with a poorer prognosis when compared to the intestinal subtype. This pattern has been confirmed as more specific markers of lower survival rates, such as the presence of signet-ring cells and poorly differentiated histology, were increasingly related to DGC.

More recently, molecular classification has added information regarding the prognostic value of DGC. In the TCGA study, the four molecular subtypes described, CIN, MSI, GS, and EBV, were not associated with significant differences in survival rates. However, ACRG data revealed that MSS-EMT patients (enriched in the DGC subtype) had the worst prognosis, after MSS-TP53$^-$, MSS-TP53$^+$, and MSI. However, in the ACRG classification, DGC was almost evenly distributed in all four subtypes. An evaluation of a larger number of DGCs might indicate differential prognosis associated with diverse mechanisms of carcinogenesis [1, 2].

In summary, important new data are beginning to unravel the carcinogenic process in DGC, further indicating that cell-adhesion and extracellular matrix processes may be disrupted in DGC. Although the incidence of the intestinal subtype has been decreasing over the years, the same is not observed for diffuse tumors. Hence, additional research is needed to unravel potential targets of therapy in DGC.

References

1. Cancer Genome Atlas Research Network. Comprehensive molecular characterization of gastric adenocarcinoma. Nature. 2014;513(7517):202–9.
2. Cristescu R, Lee J, Nebozhyn M, Kim KM, Ting JC, Wong SS, et al. Molecular analysis of gastric cancer identifies subtypes associated with distinct clinical outcomes. Nat Med. 2015;21(5):449–56.
3. Van Cutsem E, Sagaert X, Topal B, Haustermans K, Prenen H. Gastric cancer. Lancet. 2016; pii: S0140-6736(16)30354-3.
4. Forbes SA, Bhamra G, Bamford S, Dawson E, Kok C, Clements J, et al. The Catalogue of Somatic Mutations in Cancer (COSMIC). Curr Protoc Hum Genet. 2008; Chapter 10:Unit 10.11 (link accessed July 2016).
5. Wang K, Yuen ST, Xu J, Lee SP, Yan HH, Shi ST, et al. Whole-genome sequencing and comprehensive molecular profiling identify new driver mutations in gastric cancer. Nat Genet. 2014;46(6):573–82.
6. Kakiuchi M, Nishizawa T, Ueda H, Gotoh K, Tanaka A, Hayashi A, et al. Recurrent gain-of-function mutations of RHOA in diffuse-type gastric carcinoma. Nat Genet. 2014;46(6):583–7.
7. Maeda M, Ushijima T. RHOA mutation may be associated with diffuse-type gastric cancer progression, but is it gain or loss? Gastric Cancer. 2016;19(2):326–8.
8. Lee J, Lee SE, Kang SY, Do IG, Lee S, Ha SY, et al. Identification of ROS1 rearrangement in gastric adenocarcinoma. Cancer. 2013;119(9):1627–35.
9. Sharma S, Kelly TK, Jones PA. Epigenetics in cancer. Carcinogenesis. 2010;31(1):27–36.
10. Yamamoto E, Suzuki H, Takamaru H, Yamamoto H, Toyota M, Shinomura Y. Role of DNA methylation in the development of diffuse-type gastric cancer. Digestion. 2011;83(4):241–9.

11. Gigek CO, Chen ES, Calcagno DQ, Wisnieski F, Burbano RR, Smith MA. Epigenetic mechanisms in gastric cancer. Epigenomics. 2012;4(3):279–94.
12. Lin S, Gregory RI. MicroRNA biogenesis pathways in cancer. Nat Rev Cancer. 2015;15(6):321–33.
13. Yepes S, López R, Andrade RE, Rodriguez-Urrego PA, López-Kleine L, Torres MM. Co-expressed miRNAs in gastric adenocarcimona. Genomics. 2016; pii: S0888-7543(16)30071-4.
14. Dweep H, et al. miRWalk2.0: a comprehensive atlas of microRNA-target interactions. Nat Methods. 2015;12(8):697.
15. Chen J, Bardes EE, Aronow BJ, Jegga AG. ToppGene suite for gene list enrichment analysis and candidate gene prioritization. Nucleic Acids Res. 2009;37((Web Server issue)):W305–11.
16. S F, Gretschel S, Jöns T, Yashiro M, Kemmner W. THBS4, a novel stromal molecule of diffuse-type gastric adenocarcinomas, identified by transcriptome-wide expression profiling. Mod Pathol. 2011;24(10):1390–403.
17. Jinawath N, Furukawa Y, Hasegawa S, Li M, Tsunoda T, Satoh S, et al. Comparison of gene-expression profiles between diffuse- and intestinal-type gastric cancers using a genome-wide cDNA microarray. Oncogene. 2004;23(40):6830–44.
18. Bang YJ, Chung HC, Xu JM, Lordick F, Sawaki A, Lipatov O, et al. Pathological features of advanced gastric cancer: relationship to human epidermal growth factor receptor 2 positivity in the global screening programme of the ToGA trial. J Clin Oncol. 2009;27 Suppl: Abstract 4556.
19. Gall TM, Frampton AE. Gene of the month: E-cadherin (CDH1). J Clin Pathol. 2013;66(11):928–32.
20. Vinyoles M, Del Valle-Pérez B, Curto J, Viñas-Castells R, Alba-Castellón L, de Herreros G, et al. Multivesicular GSK3 sequestration upon Wnt signaling is controlled by p120-catenin/cadherin interaction with LRP5/6. Mol Cell. 2014;53(3):444–57.
21. Du W, Liu X, Fan G, Zhao X, Sun Y, Wang T, et al. From cell membrane to the nucleus: an emerging role of E-cadherin in gene transcriptional regulation. J Cell Mol Med. 2014;18(9):1712–9.
22. Kalluri R, Neilson EG. Epithelial-mesenchymal transition and its implications for fibrosis. J Clin Invest. 2003;112(12):1776–84.
23. F G, Humar B, Guilford P. The role of the E-cadherin gene (CDH1) in diffuse gastric cancer susceptibility: from the laboratory to clinical practice. Ann Oncol. 2003;14(12):1705–13.
24. Christofori G, Semb H. The role of the cell-adhesion molecule E-cadherin as a tumour-suppressor gene. Trends Biochem Sci. 1999;24(2):73–6.
25. Lazăr D, Tăban S, Ardeleanu C, Dema A, Sporea I, Cornianu M, et al. The immunohistochemical expression of E-cadherin in gastric cancer; correlations with clinicopathological factors and patients' survival. Rom J Morphol Embryol. 2008;49(4):459–67.
26. Peinado H, Portillo F, Cano A. Transcriptional regulation of cadherins during development and carcinogenesis. Int J Dev Biol. 2004;48(5–6):365–75.
27. Makdissi FB, Machado LV, Oliveira AG, Benvenuti TT, Katayama ML, Brentani MM, et al. Expression of E-cadherin, Snail and Hakai in epithelial cells isolated from the primary tumor and from peritumoral tissue of invasive ductal breast carcinomas. Braz J Med Biol Res. 2009;42(12):1128–37.
28. Aparicio LA, Valladares M, Blanco M, Alonso G, Figueroa A. Biological influence of Hakai in cancer: a 10-year. Cancer Metastasis Rev. 2012;31(1–2):375–86.
29. Suriano G, Oliveira MJ, Huntsman D, Mateus AR, Ferreira P, Casares F, Oliveira C, Carneiro F, et al. E-cadherin germline missense mutations and cell phenotype: evidence for the independence of cell invasion on the motile capabilities of the cells. Hum Mol Genet. 2003;12(22):3007–16.

Chapter 5
Genetic Predisposition and Hereditary Syndromes

Ana Carolina Ribeiro Chaves de Gouvea, Andrea Clemente Baptista Silva, Carolina Ribeiro Victor, Elizabeth Zambrano Mendoza, Mirella Nardo, and Rodrigo Santa Cruz Guindalini

Introduction

Gastric cancer (GC) is the third most common cause of death from cancer [1]. The vast majority of GCs are sporadic, but it has now been established that 1–3% of GCs arise as a result of inherited cancer predisposition syndromes [2].

These syndromes include hereditary diffuse gastric cancer (HDGC) syndrome, Li-Fraumeni syndrome, Lynch syndrome, Peutz–Jeghers syndrome, MUTYH-associated adenomatous polyposis (MAP), familial adenomatous polyposis, juvenile polyposis syndrome, and PTEN hamartoma tumor syndrome (Cowden syndrome).

Almost 20 years ago, germline mutations in the *CDH1* gene, which is responsible for encoding the protein E-cadherin, were implicated as the genetic cause of HDGC [3]. This macromolecule is a transmembrane glycoprotein expressed on epithelial tissue and is responsible for calcium-dependent cell-to-cell adhesion. E-cadherin protein is critical for establishing and maintaining polarized and differentiated epithelia through intercellular adhesion complexes. Aberrant E-cadherin activity leads to loss of cell adhesion, increased cell motility, and invasion [4]. Not only germline variants but also somatic structural alterations in *CDH1* were associated with worse prognosis and poor survival [5].

A. C. R. C. de Gouvea (✉)
Centro de Oncologia Hospital Alemao Oswaldo Cruz, São Paulo, SP, Brazil

A. C. B. Silva · C. R. Victor · E. Z. Mendoza · M. Nardo
Faculdade de Medicina da Universidade de São Paulo/Instituto do Câncer do Estado de São Paulo, São Paulo, SP, Brazil

R. S. C. Guindalini
Centro de Investigação Translacional em Oncologia, Instituto do Câncer do Estado de São Paulo, Faculdade de Medicina da Universidade de São Paulo, São Paulo, SP, Brazil

CLION, CAM Group, Salvador, Brazil

© Springer International Publishing AG, part of Springer Nature 2018
T. B. de Castria, R. S. C. Guindalini (eds.), *Diffuse Gastric Cancer*,
https://doi.org/10.1007/978-3-319-95234-5_5

41

Although considered a rare cancer predisposition syndrome, particular features in diffuse gastric cancer (DGC) patients, such as early age at diagnosis, multifocal signet-ring cell infiltrates, history of a cleft lip or cleft palate, and family history of gastric and lobular breast cancer (LBC), should call attention to the need to identify and adequately manage patients with *CDH1* germline mutations.

In this chapter, we outline clinical diagnostic criteria, indications for genetic testing, recommendations for gastric and breast cancer surveillance, and clinical and surgical management recommendations of at-risk individuals and for those carrying a *CDH1*-pathogenic mutation.

Genetic Counseling and Mutation Analysis

HDGC is a genetic syndrome with high cumulative lifetime risk of developing diffuse gastric adenocarcinoma, 70% among men and 56% among women, and lobular breast carcinoma (LBC), 39–52% among women [6, 7]. The syndrome has autosomal dominant inheritance and is correlated with a heterozygous mutation in the *CDH1* gene, a tumor suppressor gene located on chromosome 16q22.1. The association between *CDH1* pathogenic variants and HDGC was first described in New Zealand in Maori families with a strong cluster of DGC [8]; recently, an excess of LBC and oral clefts has been reported in families with HDGC [3, 9]. These recent findings led to clinical diagnostic criteria updates to help identify individuals who may benefit from genetic testing [2].

It is important that individuals who are candidates for genetic testing undergo genetic education and counseling before and after testing to facilitate informed decision making and adaptation to the risk or condition. Pretest counseling in general is associated with improvement in cancer-specific knowledge and minimal adverse psychological consequences. The risk assessment process helps individuals understand genetic testing options, their potential results, and medical implications for themselves and their relatives. Formal hereditary cancer risk assessment should access a detailed review of a three-generation family pedigree, including, if available, age at diagnosis and histology of all cancers for each family member.

The first International Gastric Cancer Linkage Consortium (IGCLC) consensus guideline, which included testing criteria for HDGC, was published in 1999 and then updated in 2010 [8, 10, 11]. According to the most recent version, published in 2015 [2], clinical criteria for the genetic screening of families with suspected hereditary GC include at least one of the criteria listed in Table 5.1.

Once a pathogenic mutation has been identified in a family, all at-risk individuals should be tested beginning at age 16–18 years [12]. Test of younger unaffected family members can be considered if there were GC cases diagnosed in earlier ages in the family.

To date, over 155 different germline *CDH1* mutations have been described, of which 126 are pathogenic and 29 are unclassified as variants of uncertain significance (VUS) [13].

Table 5.1 Clinical HDGC testing criteria

Established criteria (including first- and second-degree relatives)
2 GC cases regardless of age, at least one confirmed DGC
One case of DGC < 40 years
Personal or family history of DGC and LBC, one diagnosis < 50 years
Families in whom testing could be considered (including first- and second-degree relatives)
Bilateral LBC or family history of two or more cases of LBC < 50 years
A personal or family history of cleft lip/palate in a patient with DGC
In situ signet-ring cells or pagetoid spread of signet-ring cells

The most common mutations are frameshift mutations, insertions, and deletions (about 30% of HDGC families), followed by splice-site mutations (25%), nonsense mutations (20%), and missense mutations (20%) [14]. Large deletions account for 4% of all cases, and 1% are a result of in-frame deletions and germline promoter methylation [15]. These mutations change the expression of the E-cadherin protein, leading to a disruption of cell adhesion, incorrect binding of E-cadherin to fundamental adhesion-complex regulators, impairment of E-cadherin stability at the plasma membrane, and induction of cell migration or invasion [16].

The penetrance of GC in *CDH1* mutation carriers by age 80 years is reported to be 70% for men and 56% for women. Furthermore, the cumulative risk of LBC for women with a *CDH1* mutation is estimated to be 42% by 80 years. There is currently no evidence that the risk of other cancer types in individuals with a *CDH1* mutation is significantly increased [13].

It is recommended that carriers of a *CDH1* mutation with a desire to have children be informed about all reproductive options, including prenatal diagnosis and preimplantation genetic diagnosis.

Families meeting clinical criteria for HDGC but lacking *CDH1* mutations may harbor mutations in genes associated with other cancer predisposition syndromes. Majewski et al. reported two families with no *CDH1* mutations that were identified with germline-truncating mutations in the *CTNNA1* gene (leading to loss of α-catenin expression) [17]. Like *CDH1*, *CTNNA1* is involved in intercellular adhesion and is suspected to be a tumor suppressor and susceptibility gene for DGC. These data support the idea that germline *CTNNA1* alterations may cause HDGC and should be considered in the screening of prospective families.

Screening and Surveillance

Endoscopic Screening for Gastric Cancer

The guidelines consider that individuals with unknown mutation status or without proven pathogenic *CDH1* mutation should undergo annual standardized endoscopic screening for GC.

Individuals who tested positive for a pathogenic germline *CDH1* mutation should be advised to consider prophylactic gastrectomy, regardless of endoscopic findings. Nevertheless, prophylactic gastrectomy is an unacceptable option for many mutation carriers due to early and late potential medical or psychosocial complications. As an alternative, mutation carriers should be offered the option of annual endoscopy surveillance with a strict protocol with visual inspection followed by random biopsy sampling.

Endoscopy with biopsy sampling aims to detect microscopic foci of intramucosal signet-ring cell carcinoma and its precursor lesions and should be performed at centers with experienced endoscopists and gastrointestinal pathologist [2]. The biopsies should include sampling of any visible lesions and at least six random biopsies from each of the five anatomical zones (antrum, transitional zone, body, fundus, cardia) [10]. It is recommended that these individuals undergo screening every 6–12 months beginning 5–10 years before the earliest cancer diagnosis in the family [8, 18].

It might be useful to follow these recommendations:

1. Stop the anticoagulants (e.g., Warfarin, clopidogrel) because the bleeding risk might be slightly higher than for other indications since more biopsies are taken.
2. Before an examination, wash the mucosa with a combination of mucolytics (N-acetylcysteine) and antifoaming agent (such as simethicone) mixed with sterile water.
3. Use a white-light, high-definition endoscope in a dedicated session of at least 30 min to allow for careful inspection of the mucosa on repeated inflation and deflation and for the collection of biopsies.
4. Record the macroscopic appearances of the gastric mucosa and any focal visible lesions, using still images or video for future reference and specifically sampled for histology prior to the collection of random biopsies.
5. Inflate and deflate the stomach, prior to examination for small *foci*, to check distensibility.

Due to the small *foci* of signet-ring cells, a biopsy of any endoscopically visible lesions, including pale areas, is recommended using a standard forceps with a spike to include lamina propria cells. This is required to maximize the likelihood of diagnosing microscopic alterations [2].

The experience of pathologists and the accuracy of diagnosis have improved. The use of periodic acid-Schiff (PAS) and diastase digestion may be useful for the detection or confirmation of small intramucosal carcinomas. E-cadherin immunoexpression has been shown to reduce or be absent in early invasive gastric carcinomas of mutation carriers. However, its expression may vary depending on the mutation site and specific mechanisms of inactivation of the wild-type allele [2, 10].

All patients undergoing endoscopy surveillance for HDGC should be informed that, given the very focal and often endoscopically invisible nature of these lesions, it is quite possible that lesions will not be detected by random biopsies.

Breast Cancer Surveillance

Women who carry pathogenic *CDH1* gene mutations have an additional 40% risk of developing LBC. Therefore, breast cancer surveillance is recommended. Because of limited data, the breast cancer surveillance guidelines are based on those for women with a *BRCA1* or *BRCA2* mutation.

LBC is characterized histologically by small cells that infiltrate along and around ducts in single file without destroying the underlying architecture and typically does not induce a desmoplastic reaction. Moreover, staining for E-cadherin is typically not expressed with a consequent loss of cohesion of tumor cells and susceptibility to a pervasive growth pattern [19]. Because of these histological features – not creating a substantial reaction in connective tissues or destroying other anatomical structures – LBC can be hard to spot on a mammogram. The sensitivity of mammography to lobular carcinoma varies between 64% and 92%. Given the reduced radiodensity and low presence or absence of suspicious microcalcifications, mammography may be normal in 30% of cases, with a false negative rate oscillating between 19 and 66% [20].

The three-dimensional mammogram (tomosynthesis) seems to have greater sensitivity than the digital mammography in identifying such tumors; however, the available published data in this regard are insufficient, and further studies are needed. Today, breast magnetic resonance imaging (MRI) seems to be the method of choice for the assessment of infiltrating lobular carcinoma. It is more sensitive in identifying tumors, assessing the extension and presence of multiple or contralateral foci, and modifying surgery in 28.3% of cases [21]. Therefore, annual breast MRI is recommended for breast cancer screening for women with *CDH1* mutations starting at age 30. MRI can be combined with mammography [2].

Gastrectomy and Mastectomy

Prophylactic Gastrectomy: Indications for and Timing of Surgery

Prophylactic gastrectomy should be recommended in carriers of pathogenic germline *CDH1* mutation. Some experts believe that the best term in this context is *risk reduction gastrectomy* because the majority of mutation carriers already have microscopic signet-ring cell carcinomas at the time of their surgery (at least T1a cancers) [2].

Total gastrectomy for these patients, however, completely eliminates their risk of GC and is truly prophylactic in terms of preventing their death from invasive GC.

The optimal timing of prophylactic gastrectomy is unknown and is usually highly individualized. Since this surgery has a major impact on the quality of life, the decision to undergo prophylactic gastrectomy should be well informed, balanced, prepared, and timed. Decisional counseling, weighing the pros and cons of intervention, is essential. The current consensus is that the procedure should be discussed and offered in early adulthood, generally between 20 and 30 years of age, and family phenotype, particularly the age of onset of GC in probands, should be taken into account to determine the most appropriate time.

Before the surgery, a baseline endoscopy should be performed to look for macroscopic tumors, as this may alter the treatment plan. The recommended surgery is total gastrectomy with Roux-en-Y reconstruction [2].

The optimal extent of lymph node dissection (LND) in prophylactic gastrectomy is controversial. Lymph node disseminations are not reported in asymptomatic *CDH1* mutation carriers with negative preoperative endoscopic screening biopsies. The frequency of lymph node metastasis increases according to the size and the stage; in pT1a tumors, it is 2–5% [22], and in pT1b tumors, with invasion of the submucosal layer, lymph node metastases are found in 17–28% in cases [23]. Because a preoperative gastroduodenoscopy cannot exclude the presence of T1b lesions with their higher risk of metastases during the operation, a D1 LND (with the inclusion of lymph node stations 1–7) is reasonable.

Gastrectomy induces in patients several psychological, physiological, and metabolic injuries that should not be underestimated. Most patients will return to an active life after their operation, and the global quality of life to presurgery levels will recover at around 12 months postoperatively [24].

There are no established programs for recovery post gastrectomy, but patients will require the support of a multidisciplinary team for adjustments to diet, caloric intake, vitamin supplementation, hydration, behavior modifications with respect to eating, and anatomical changes. It is necessary to discuss with patients all treatment options to improve recovery progress [2].

Prophylactic Mastectomy

Prophylactic mastectomy is not routinely recommended but may be a reasonable option for some women. No specific data address this procedure in this population, and evidence from BRCA1/2 carriers can be used and discussed with each patient.

In summary, the current guideline proposes the following management for patients with HDGC [25] (Table 5.2).

It is important to highlight that recent studies have found patients with *CDH1* mutations that do not have a family or personal history of gastric or breast cancer. In this scenario, the benefit of invasive approaches like prophylactic surgeries has not yet been established [10]. Therefore, more information about *CDH1* mutation penetrance is needed to improve counseling of asymptomatic families in order to avoid unnecessary procedures.

Table 5.2 Summary recommendation for management of patients with *CDH1* germline pathogenic mutations

Prophylactic gastrectomy after 20 years of age
Breast cancer surveillance in women beginning at age 30 years with annual mammography and breast MRI and clinical breast examination every 6 months
Colonoscopy beginning at age 40 years for families with a history of colon cancer (conditional recommendation, low quality of evidence).

References

1. Ferlay J, Soerjomataram I, & Ervik M, et al. GLOBOCAN 2012 v1.0, Cancer incidence and mortality worldwide: IARC cancer base no. 11 [Internet]. International Agency for Research on Cancer, Lyon, 2014.
2. Van der Post RS, Vogelaar IP, Carmeorp F, et al. Hereditary diffuse gastric cancer: updated clinical guidelines with an emphasis on germline CDH1 mutation carriers. J Med Genet. 2015;52:361–74.
3. Guilford P, Hopkins J, Harraway J, et al. E-cadherin germline mutations in familial gastric cancer. Nature. 1998;392:402–5.
4. Takeichi M, Hirano S, Matsuyoshi N, Fujimori T. Cytoplasmic control of cadherin-mediated cell-cell adhesion. Cold Spring Harb Symp Quant Biol. 1992;57:327–34.
5. Corso G, Carvalho J, Marrelli D, Vindigni C, Carvalho B, Seruca R, Roviello F, Oliveira C. Somatic mutations and deletions of the E-cadherin gene predict poor survival of patients with gastric cancer. J Clin Oncol. 2013;31(7):868–75. https://doi.org/10.1200/JCO.2012.44.4612. Epub 2013 Jan 22.
6. Guilford P, Humar B, Blair V. Hereditary diffuse gastric cancer: translation of CDH1 germline mutations into clinical practice. Gastric Cancer. 2010;13:1–10.
7. Kaurah P, MacMillan A, Boyd N, et al. Founder and recurrent CDH1 mutations in families with hereditary diffuse gastric cancer. JAMA. 2007;297:2360–72.
8. Caldas C, Carneiro F, Lynch HT, Yokota J, Wiesner GL, Powell SM, Lewis FR, Huntsman DG, Pharoah PD, Jankowski JA, MacLeod P, Vogelsang H, Keller G, Park KG, Richards FM, Maher ER, Gayther SA, Oliveira C, Grehan N, Wight D, Seruca R, Roviello F, Ponder BA, Jackson CE. Familial gastric cancer: overview and guidelines for management. J Med Genet. 1999;36:873–80.
9. Brito LA, Yamamoto GL, Melo S, Malcher C, Ferreira SG, Figueiredo J, Alvizi L, Kobayashi GS, Naslavsky MS, Alonso N, Feliz TM, Zatz M, Seruca R, Passos Bueno MR. Rare variants in the epithelial cadherin gene underlying the genetic etiology of nonsyndromic cleft lip with or without cleft palate. Hum Mutat. 2015;36(11):1029–33. https://doi.org/10.1002/humu.22827.
10. Fitzgerald RC, Hardwick R, Huntsman D, Carneiro F, Guilford P, Blair V, Chung DC, Norton J, Ragunath K, Van Krieken JH, Dwerryhouse S, Caldas C, International Gastric Cancer Linkage Consortium. Hereditary diffuse gastric cancer: updated consensus guidelines for clinical management and directions for future research. J Med Genet. 2010;47:436–44.
11. Mouret-Fourme E, Noguès C, Di Maria M, Tlemsani C, Warcoin M, Grandjouan S, Malka D, Caron O, Blayau M. Hereditary diffuse gastric cancer syndrome: improved performances of the 2015 testing criteria for the identification of probands with a CDH1 germline mutation. J Med Genet. 2015;52(8):563–5.
12. Blair V, Martin I, Shaw D, et al. Hereditary diffuse gastric cancer: diagnosis and management. Clin Gastroenterol Hepatol. 2006;4:262–75.

13. Hansford S, Kaurah P, Li-Chang H, Woo M, Senz J, Pinheiro H, Schrader KA, Schaeffer DF, Shumansky K, Zogopoulos G, Almeida Santos T, Claro I, Carvalho J, Nielsen C, Padilla S, Lum A, Talhouk A, Baker-Lange K, Richardson S, Lewis I, Lindor NM, Pennell E, MacMillan A, Fernandez B, Keller G, Lynch H, Shah SP, Guilford P, Gallinger S, Corso G, Roviello F, Caldas C, Oliveria C, Pharoah PDP, Huntsman DG. Hereditary diffuse gastric cancer syndrome: CDH1 mutations and beyond. JAMA Oncol. 2015;1:23.
14. Oliveira C, Senz J, Kaurah P, et al. Germline CDH1 deletions in hereditary diffuse gastric cancer families. Hum Mol Genet. 2009;18:1545–55.
15. Oliveira C, Seruca R, Hoogerbrugge N, et al. Clinical utility gene card for: hereditary diffuse gastric cancer (HDGC). Eur J Hum Genet. 2013;21(8):e1–5 [Epub ahead of print].
16. Humar B, Guilford P. Hereditary diffuse gastric cancer: a manifestation of lost cell polarity. Cancer Sci. 2009;100:1151–7.
17. Majewski IJ, Kluijt I, Cats A, et al. An α-E-catenin (CTNNA1) mutation in hereditary diffuse gastric cancer. J Pathol. 2013;229(4):621–9.
18. Brooks-Wilson AR, Kaurah P, Suriano G, et al. Germline E-cadherin mutations in hereditary diffuse gastric cancer: assessment of 42 new families and review of genetic screening criteria. J Med Genet. 2004;41:508–17.
19. Moll R, Mitze M, Frixen UH, Birchmeier W. Differential loss of E-cadherin expression in infiltrating ductal and lobular breast carcinomas. Am J Pathol. 1993;143(6):1731–42.
20. Brem RF, Ioffe M, Rapelyea JA, Yost KG, Weigert JM, Bertrand ML, Stern LH. Invasive lobular carcinoma: detection with mammography, sonography, MRI, and breast-specific gamma imaging. AJR Am J Roentgenol. 2009;192(2):379–83.
21. Oliveira TM, Elias J Jr, Melo AF, Teixeira SR, Filho SC, Gonçalves LM, Faria FM, Tiezzi DG, Andrade JM, Muglia V. Evolving concepts in breast lobular neoplasia and invasive lobular carcinoma, and their impact on imaging methods. Insights Imaging. 2014;5(2):183–94.
22. Gotoda T, Yanagisawa A, Sasako M, Ono H, Nakanishi Y, Shimoda T, Kato Y. Incidence of lymph node metastasis from early gastric cancer: estimation with a 99 large number of cases at two large centers. Gastric Cancer. 2000;3:219–25.
23. Roviello F, Rossi S, Marrelli D, Pedrazzani C, Corso G, Vindigni C, Morgagni P, Saragoni L, de Manzoni G, Tomezzoli A. Number of lymph node metastases and its prognostic significance in early gastric cancer: a multicenter Italian study. J Surg Oncol. 2006;94:275–80; discussion 4.
24. Muir J, Aronson M, Esplen MJ, Pollett A, Swallow CJ. Prophylactic Total gastrectomy: a prospective cohort study of long-term impact on quality of life. J Gastrointest Surg. 2016;20(12):1950–8. Epub 2016 Oct 17.
25. Syngal S, Brand RE, Church JM, Giardiello FM, Hampel HL, Burt RW. ACG clinical guideline: genetic testing and management of hereditary gastrointestinal cancer syndromes. Am J Gastroenterol. 2015;110:223–62.

Chapter 6
The Role of Surgery

Ulysses Ribeiro Jr. and Fernando Simionato Perrotta

Management of Primary Tumor Site

Despite multimodal gastric cancer (GC) treatment, the role of surgery is the central pillar in treatment. The principles of surgical treatment differ only regarding the margin in diffuse gastric cancer (DGC). Surgical planning will be guided by preoperative staging. Early GCs (T1a) can be managed with endoscopic resection through endoscopic mucosal resection (EMR) or endoscopic submucosal dissection (ESD), the latter technique being the most recommended. However, the classic criteria for endoscopic resection include only the well-differentiated carcinomas, and this therapeutic modality is still considered investigational for undifferentiated tumors. The expanded criteria for undifferentiated-type (only ESD should be employed) are tumors clinically diagnosed as T1a, ≤ 2 cm in diameter, and without ulceration [1]. T1 tumors that do not meet the criteria for endoscopic resection should be treated surgically. For those who do not have positive lymph nodes, a macroscopic margin of at least 2 cm should be obtained [1–4]. For T1b tumors with no positive lymph node, standard treatment consists of total or subtotal gastrectomy followed by D1 lymphadenectomy. The standard surgical treatment for tumors with positive lymph node or T2-T4a consists of total or subtotal gastrectomy associated with D2 lymphadenectomy. In this scenario, for DGC, a greater surgical margin is recommended. Its diffusely invasive growth pattern makes it difficult for surgeons to macroscopically ensure a cancer-free margin [3].

U. Ribeiro Jr. (✉)
University of São Paulo School of Medicine, Instituto do Câncer do Estado de São Paulo, ICESP-HCFMUSP, São Paulo, SP, Brazil
e-mail: Ulysses.ribeiro@fm.usp.br

F. S. Perrotta
Department of Gastroenterology, University of São Paulo School of Medicine, São Paulo, SP, Brazil

© Springer International Publishing AG, part of Springer Nature 2018
T. B. de Castria, R. S. C. Guindalini (eds.), *Diffuse Gastric Cancer*,
https://doi.org/10.1007/978-3-319-95234-5_6

49

The positive surgical margin is an isolated factor of poor prognosis after surgical treatment and is related to a more aggressive tumor biology, which is related to DGC. A study conducted in Taiwan involving 1565 GC patients showed that 1421 patients undergoing gastrectomy with negative margin had a 3-, 5-, and 9-year overall survival (OS) rate of 66.8%, 60.0%, and 53.3%, respectively. However, GC patients undergoing gastrectomy with positive microscopic resection had 3-, 5-, and 9-year OS rates of 24.0%, 13.4%, and 11.5%, respectively [5]. Another study with 2728 patients conducted in China revealed a significantly lower 5-year survival rate in patients with positive margins compared to patients with negative margins (25.8% vs. 52.6%, $P = 0.001$). The diffuse type showed a correlation with the positivity of the surgical margins [6]. In a historical series of cases from the Memorial Sloan-Kettering Cancer Center involving 2384 patients, there was a higher frequency of positive surgical margin in the diffuse histotype (54% margin compromised vs. 29% free margin) [7]. For the reasons discussed, for the diffuse histotype with positive lymph nodes or T2-T4a, a surgical margin of 7–8 cm is recommended [2, 4]. If this margin cannot be obtained, the total gastrectomy is indicated. As an alternative in cases with difficulty in establishing surgical margin, intraoperative frozen section may be performed. However, a frozen section used in the evaluation of margins may produce false negatives. A study conducted to evaluate margins through frozen section and to amplify them when positive demonstrated no improved recurrence-free survival (RFS) and OS, only a decrease in local recurrence [8].

Another important surgical aspect related to DGC is the higher risk of peritoneal recurrence, especially in the presence of gastric serosa invasion. This aspect must have clinical relevance during the surgical procedure [9].

The peritoneal surface is the most common site of GC recurrence after surgery. After curative resection, peritoneal dissemination may occur in 20–50% of cases and rises up to 80% in cases with positive peritoneal cytology [10]. The problem is that adjuvant intravenous chemotherapy or radiotherapy does not improve survival in patients at high risk of peritoneal dissemination. Only intraperitoneal chemotherapy may prevent the development of peritoneal dissemination, and the addition of hyperthermia synergistically with some drugs may increase the depth of penetration into the tissue [11]. Other possible delivery options have been described, including perioperative normothermic intraperitoneal chemotherapy (NIPEC), hyperthermic intraperitoneal chemotherapy (HIPEC), early postoperative intraperitoneal chemotherapy (EPIC), and delayed postoperative intraperitoneal chemotherapy (DIPEC) [12, 13].

Initial intraperitoneal chemotherapy studies demonstrated that patients receiving chemotherapy intraperitoneally with mitomycin C, but also cisplatin and 5-FU, had better overall survival after curative resection of locally advanced GC [14].

One study with 107 patients treated with HIPEC revealed that patients who underwent complete resection had better 5-year survival than those with residual peritoneal disease (13% vs. 2%) [15].

Two meta-analyses examined intraperitoneal chemotherapy. Xu et al. [16] analyzed 11 randomized clinical trials, 7 comparing surgery + HIPEC vs. surgery alone.

Intraperitoneal chemotherapy was superior after curative surgery vs. surgery alone, and a combination of HIPEC and activated carbon particles was significantly better than other drug combinations. The second meta-analysis, by Yan et al. [17], reviewed all clinical trials of intraperitoneal chemotherapy. Among 13 trials, 4 investigated the efficacy of HIPEC, 5 NIPEC, 2 EPIC, 2 combined HIPEC and EPIC, and finally, 2 trials reported the combined effects of DIPEC. All data from 1648 patients showed a significant difference in survival of patients treated with HIPEC, or HIPEC together with EPIC. A trend toward survival improvement was observed with NIPEC. No benefit was seen using EPIC or DIPEC.

A new trial is ongoing to prove the effectiveness of HIPEC during curative gastrectomy in the case of positive peritoneal cytology (GASTRICHIP trial). Perhaps in the future this technique can be applied to reduce the peritoneal recurrence in DGC [13].

Lymphadenectomy

DGC is associated with a higher risk of lymph node metastasis even in the early stages, which demands an extensive lymphadenectomy [9]. A study conducted in Japan involving 316 GC patients – 153 diffuse and 163 intestinal type – demonstrated lymph node metastasis in 84 (54.9%) and 45 (27.6%), respectively, showing the highest incidence of lymph node metastasis in the diffuse histotype [18].

The various guidelines for the treatment of GC do not take into account the histotype to determine the type of lymphadenectomy to be used. The type of lymphadenectomy to be employed is determined by the stage according to the the Union for International Cancer Control (UICC)/American Joint Committee on Cancer (AJCC) TNM classification. The size (T) and lymph node status (N) of the tumor are considered to define the type of lymphadenectomy to be employed. The different types of lymphadenectomy are classified according to the resected lymph node chains. In general, D1 or D1 + lymphadenectomy is indicated for cT1N0 tumors and D2 for positive node or cT2-T4 tumors. Lymph node dissection for T1 tumors should be limited to perigastric lymph nodes (with variation in nodal groups dissected according to the tumor site, which should be designated by D1, followed by the number of the extra chain dissected). The D2 lymphadenectomy implies the removal of perigastric lymph nodes plus those along the left gastric, common hepatic, and splenic arteries and the celiac axis [1, 2, 4].

The Japanese guideline provides details about the lymph nodes to be resected based not only on the T and N but also on the location of the lesion in the stomach. American and European consensus specifies, not the lymph node chains to be resected, but the total number of resected lymph nodes. A minimum of 15 lymph nodes should be present in a D2 lymphadenectomy. Other guidelines recommend a greater number of lymph nodes resection, reaching up to a minimum of 25 lymph nodes [19, 20].

Surgical Access

Laparoscopy

Laparoscopic access for the treatment of GC can be considered for distal and early tumors [1, 2, 4]. Large studies have been conducted to examine noninferiority in relation to oncologic outcomes compared to conventional access for the treatment of GC. Trials are currently ongoing in Japan (JCOG), Korea (KLASS-02), and China to compare open versus laparoscopic surgery in GC, and these should provide further evidence regarding the role of laparoscopic surgery. The histological type has not been taken into account for the indication of laparoscopic access in GC. The main aspects to consider when recruiting patients to trials involving laparoscopic gastrectomy (LG) versus open gastrectomy (OG) are locoregional staging, tumor location, and type of surgery required for treatment (total gastrectomy × subtotal). The greatest evidence for laparoscopic surgery was demonstrated for the initial distal GCs that require less extensive lymphadenectomies and subtotal gastrectomy. The Korean KLASS-01 phase 3 prospective, multicenter, controlled study comparing LG and OG, for example, did not specify the histological subtype in the inclusion criteria [21]. A randomized controlled trial from the Chinese Laparoscopic Gastrointestinal Surgery Study (CLASS) designed to compare laparoscopic distal gastrectomy (LDG) and open distal gastrectomy (ODG) with D2 lymph node dissections for advanced GC enrolled a total of 1039 (519 patients in the laparoscopic gastrectomy group and 520 patients in the open gastrectomy group). The compliance rates of D2 lymphadenectomy were similar between the LG and OG groups (99.4% vs. 99.6%; $P = 0.845$). However, the resection margin was considerably smaller in LG. In the LDG group, the mean proximal margin was 4.8 cm and the mean distal margin was 4.1 cm. In comparison, in the ODG group, the mean proximal margin was 5.2 cm and the mean distal margin was 4.3 cm. Postoperative morbidity and mortality were similar between the two groups. This difference regarding the surgical margin could have some impact on oncologic outcome for DGC, particularly in advanced GC. Long-term results analysis could show better evidence for laparoscopic access for DGC [22]. At present, trials are showing the same oncologic outcomes in OG and LG, even at the advanced stage. But more consistent data are needed.

Prophylactic Gastrectomy in Hereditary Diffuse Gastric Cancer

The vast majority of GCs are sporadic, but it has now been established that 1–3% of GCs arise as a result of inherited cancer predisposition syndromes. Historically, hereditary diffuse gastric cancer (HDGC) syndrome is characterized by a germline mutation in the *CDH1* tumor suppressor gene encoding the E-caderin protein.

E-caderin is a transmembrane glycoprotein that mediates calcium-dependent cellular adhesion and is important for cell polarity and epithelial differentiation during development. This mutation is identified in 30–50% of cases of HDGC and is related to an increased risk of DGC and lobular carcinoma of the breast at an early age. Because not all cases in which HDGC is characterized is such a mutation present, other genes are also involved in its predisposition, and some of them are described as a mutation in the *CTNNA1* gene [23–26].

Genetic testing for *CDH1* mutations should be considered when any of the following criteria are met: (1) two GC cases in one family, one confirmed case of DGC diagnosed before age 50 years; (2) three confirmed cases of DGC in first- or second-degree relative independent of age; (3) DGC diagnosed before age 40 years without a family history; or (4) personal or family history of DGC and lobular breast cancer, one diagnosed before age 50 years [27].

Early endoscopic detection of these lesions is still flawed; therefore, it should not be considered standard recommendation. Prophylactic gastrectomy is recommended between the ages of 18 and 40 for patients with the mutation in the *CDH1* gene. It can be considered before age 18 for patients with relatives who were diagnosed with GC before the age of 25. A total gastrectomy should be performed and the proximal and distal margin should be sent to frozen section analysis. The proximal margin should confirm columnar squamous esophageal epithelium, and the distal margin should confirm duodenal epithelium, in order to eliminate the possibility of leaving gastric epithelium unremoved. Lymphadenectomy is controversial. In general, it is not recommended; however, some patients, even if asymptomatic, may already present diffuse adenocarcinoma with a risk of lymph node metastasis, although in a small percentage. Thus, it would be reasonable to consider D1 lymphadenectomy for these patients (inclusion of lymph nodes from stations 1 to 7) since this procedure does not significantly increase the morbidity and mortality of gastrectomy [27, 28].

Diffuse Gastric Cancer in Young Patients

DGC in young patients is thought to exhibit a worse prognosis owing to specific clinicopathologic characteristics and delayed diagnosis; however, the data are controversial. Some studies have shown that patients aged 40 years or younger with DGC exhibited a predominance of females, diffuse stomach lesions, signet-ring cell type, poorly differentiated histological tumors, Borrmann type IV, mixed Lauren's classification type, and high recurrence rate in the gastric remnant. However, the overall 5-year survival rate may be better than among older patients, stratifying by stage at diagnosis [29, 30].

Diffuse Gastric Cancer and Prognosis

DGC is generally thought to have a worse prognosis and lower chemosensitivity than non-signet-ring cancer cell (SRCC). However, the prognosis of SRCC and its chemosensitivity with specific regimens are still controversial because SRCC is not specifically identified in most studies and its poor prognosis may be due to its more advanced stage.

In the USA, relative 5-year survival rates for GC increased from 15–29% during the period 1975–2009. However, GC survival remains poor. Cardia GC and diffuse-type noncardia GC present with the worst prognosis [31]. Compared to tumors in the pyloric antrum, cardia GC patients have lower 5-year survival rates and higher operative mortality [32, 33].

Conclusions

DGC is an aggressive histotype and must be treated accordingly. Endoscopic resection should be reserved for mucosal lesions smaller than 2 cm without ulcerations. Early tumors larger than that should be referred to surgical resection, open or minimally invasive. Advanced tumors are better treated by resection with an extensive margin of at least 7 cm and D2 lymphadenectomy.

Intraoperative chemotherapy has been tested to verify its role in the treatment and prevention of peritoneal recurrence. Nonetheless, efforts should be made to improve the prognosis of DGC patients.

References

1. Japanese Gastric Cancer Association. Japanese gastric cancer treatment guidelines 2014 (ver. 4). Gastric Cancer. 2017;20:1–19.
2. De Manzoni G, Marrelli D, Baiocchi GL, Morgagni P, Saragoni L, Degiuli M, Donini A, Fumagalli U, Mazzei MA, Pacelli F. The Italian Research Group for Gastric Cancer (GIRCG) guidelines for gastric cancer staging and treatment: 2015. Gastric Cancer. 2017;20:20–30.
3. Fitzgerald RC, Hardwick R, Huntsman D, Carneiro F, Guilford P, Blair V, Chung DC, Norton J, Ragunath K, Van Krieken JH, Dwerryhouse S, Caldas C, International Gastric Cancer Linkage C. Hereditary diffuse gastric cancer: updated consensus guidelines for clinical management and directions for future research. J Med Genet. 2010;47:436–44.
4. Smyth EC, Verheij M, Allum W, Cunningham D, Cervantes A, Anold D, on behalf of the ESMO Guidelines Committe. Gastric cancer: ESMO Clinical Practice Guidelines for diagnosis, treatment and follow-up. Annals of Oncology. 2016;27(Supplement 5):v38–49. https://doi.org/10.1093/annonc/mdw350.
5. Wang SY, Yeh CN, Lee HL, et al. Clinical impact of positive surgical margin status on gastric cancer patients undergoing gastrectomy. Ann Surg Oncol. 2009;16:2738–43.
6. Sun Z, Li DM, Wang ZN, et al. Prognostic significance of microscopic positive margins for gastric cancer patients with potentially curative resection. Ann Surg Oncol. 2009;16:3028–37.

7. Bickenbach KA, Gonen M, Strong V, Brennan MF, Coit DG. Association of positive transection margins with gastric cancer survival and local recurrence. Ann Surg Oncol. 2013;20:2663–8.
8. Squires MH 3rd, Kooby DA, Pawlik DA, et al. Utility of the proximal margin frozen section for resection of gastric adenocarcinoma: a 7-institution study of the US Gastric Cancer Collaborative. Ann Surg Oncol. 2014;21:4202–10.
9. Marrelli D, Pedrazzani C, Morgagni P, de Manzoni G, Pacelli F, Coniglio A, et al. Italian Research Group for Gastric Cancer. Changing clinical and pathological features of gastric cancer over time. Br J Surg. 2011;98:1273–83.
10. Shen P, Stewart JH, Levine EA. Cytoreductive surgery and hyperthermic intraperitoneal chemotherapy for peritoneal surface malignancy: overview and rationale. Curr Probl Cancer. 2009;33:125–41.
11. Roviello F, Caruso S, Neri A, Marrelli D. Treatment and prevention of peritoneal carcinomatosis from gastric cancer by cytoreductive surgery and hyperthermic intraperitoneal chemotherapy: overview and rationale. Eur J Surg Oncol. 2013;39:1309–16.
12. Glehen O, Gilly FN, Arvieux C, Cotte E, Boutitie F, Mansvelt B, Bereder JM, Lorimier G, Quenet F, Elias D. Peritoneal carcinomatosis from gastric cancer: a multi-institutional study of 159 patients treated by cytoreductive surgery combined with perioperative intraperitoneal chemotherapy. Ann Surg Oncol. 2010;17:2370–7.
13. Marrelli D, Polom K, de Manzoni G, Morgagni P, Baiocchi GL, Roviello F. Multimodal treatment of gastric cancer in the west: where are we going? World J Gastroenterol. 2015;21(26):7954–69.
14. Bozzetti F, Yu W, Baratti D, Kusamura S, Deraco M. Locoregional treatment of peritoneal carcinomatosis from gastric cancer. J Surg Oncol. 2008;98:273–6.
15. Yonemura Y, Kawamura T, Bandou E, Takahashi S, Sawa T, Matsuki N. Treatment of peritoneal dissemination from gastric cancer by peritonectomy and chemohyperthermic peritoneal perfusion. Br J Surg. 2005;92:370–5.
16. Xu DZ, Zhan YQ, Sun XW, Cao SM, Geng QR. Meta-analysis of intraperitoneal chemotherapy for gastric cancer. World J Gastroenterol. 2004;10:2727–30.
17. Yan TD, Black D, Sugarbaker PH, Zhu J, Yonemura Y, Petrou G, Morris DL. A systematic review and meta-analysis of the randomized controlled trials on adjuvant intraperitoneal chemotherapy for resectable gastric cancer. Ann Surg Oncol. 2007;14:2702–13.
18. Zheng H, Takahashi H, Murai Y, Cui Z, Nomoto K, Miwa S, Tsuneyama K, Takano Y. Pathobiological characteristics of intestinal and diffuse-type gastric carcinoma in Japan: an immunostaining study on the tissue microarray. J Clin Pathol. 2006;60:273–7.
19. Zilberstein B, Malheiros C, Lourenço LG, Kassab P, Jacob CE, Weston AC, Bresciani CJC, Castro O, Gama-Rodrigues J, de Consenso G. Consenso brasileiro sobre câncer gástrico: diretrizes para o câncer gástrico no Brasil. ABCD Arq Bras Cir Dig. 2013;26(1):2–6.
20. Moehler M, Baltin CTH, Ebert M, Fischbach W, Gockel I, Grenacher L, et al. International comparison of the German evidence-based S3-guidelines on the diagnosis and multimodal treatment of early and locally advanced gastric cancer, including adenocarcinoma of the lower esophagus. Gastric Cancer. 2015;18:550–63.
21. Kim W, Kim HH, Han SU, et al. Decreased morbidity of laparoscopic distal gastrectomy compared with open distal gastrectomy for stage I gastric cancer: short-term outcomes from a multicenter randomized controlled trial (KLASS-01). Ann Surg. 2016;263:28–35.
22. Hu Y, Huang C, Sun Y, et al. Morbidity and mortality of laparoscopic versus open D2 distal gastrectomy for advanced gastric cancer: a randomized controlled trial. J Clin Oncol. 2016;34:1350–7. https://doi.org/10.1200/JCO.2015.63.7215.
23. Takeichi M. Morphogenetic roles of classic cadherins. Curr Opin Cell Biol. 1995;7:619–27.
24. Geisbrecht ER, Montell DJ. Myosin VI is required for E-cadherin-mediated border cell migration. Nat Cell Biol. 2002;4:616–20.
25. Machado JC, Oliveira C, Carvalho R, et al. E-cadherin gene (CDH1) promoter methylation as the second hit in sporadic diffuse gastric carcinoma. Oncogene. 2001;20:1525–8.

26. Berx G, Cleton-Jansen AM, Nollet F, et al. E-cadherin is a tumour/invasion suppressor gene mutated in human lobular breast cancers. EMBO J. 1995;14:6107–15.
27. van der Post RS, Vogelaar IP, Carneiro F, et al. Hereditary diffuse gastric cancer: updated clinical guidelines with an emphasis on germline CDH1 mutation carriers. J Med Genet. 2015;52:361–74.
28. Chen Y, Kingham K, Ford JM, et al. A prospective study of total gastrectomy for CDH1-positive hereditary diffuse gastric cancer. Ann Surg Oncol. 2011;18:2594–8.
29. Wang Z, Xu J, Shi Z, Shen X, Luo T, Bi J, Nie M. Clinicopathologic characteristics and prognostic of gastric cancer in young patients. Scand J Gastroenterol. 2016;51(9):1043–9.
30. Pernot S, Voron T, Perkins G, Lagorce-Pages C, Berger A, Taieb J. Signet-ring cell carcinoma of the stomach: impact on prognosis and specific therapeutic challenge. World J Gastroenterol. 2015;21(40):11428–38.
31. Crew KD, Neugut AI. Epidemiology of gastric cancer. World J Gastroenterol. 2006;12(3):354–62.
32. Dassen AE, Lemmens VE, van de Poll-Franse LV, et al. Trends in incidence, treatment and survival of gastric adenocarcinoma between 1990 and 2007: a population-based study in the Netherlands. Eur J Cancer. 2010;46(6):1101–10.
33. Marqués-Lespier JM, González-Pons M, Cruz-Correa M. Current perspectives on gastric Cancer. Gastroenterol Clin N Am. 2016;45(3):413–28.

Chapter 7
The Role of Radiation Therapy

Andre Tsin Chih Chen and Carlos Bo Chur Hong

Abbreviations

5-FU + LV	5-fluorouracil plus leucovorin
CMT	Chemotherapy
CRT	Chemoradiation
CT	Computerized tomography
DFS	Disease-free survival
Gy	Gray
HR	Hazard ratio
OR	Odds ratio
OS	Overall survival
RFS	Relapse-free survival
RT	Radiation therapy
XP	Capecitabine and cisplatin
XRT	Capecitabine with radiation therapy

Most patients with gastric cancer will have a locoregional failure after surgery alone [1]. The purpose of adjuvant RT is to achieve locoregional control that will ultimately translate into a survival benefit. In 2001, Macdonald et al. published the results of the Gastrointestinal Cancer Intergroup 0116 (INT 0116), setting CRT as the standard treatment of resected gastric cancer in Western countries [2].

A. T. C. Chen (✉)
Instituto do Câncer do Estado de São Paulo, São Paulo, SP, Brazil
e-mail: andre.chen@hc.fm.usp.br

C. B. C. Hong
Faculdade de Medicina da Universidade de São Paulo/Instituto do Câncer
do Estado de São Paulo, São Paulo, SP, Brazil

© Springer International Publishing AG, part of Springer Nature 2018
T. B. de Castria, R. S. C. Guindalini (eds.), *Diffuse Gastric Cancer*,
https://doi.org/10.1007/978-3-319-95234-5_7

INT 0116

The INT 0116 randomized 556 patients to surgery alone or surgery plus adjuvant CRT. Adjuvant treatment consisted of a 5-day cycle of fluorouracil and leucovorin (5-FU + LV) followed by concurrent CRT starting on D28 (45 Gy in 25 fractions plus concurrent 5-FU + LV, 4 days/week at the beginning and at the end of radiation). After completing CRT, two additional 5-day cycles of 5-FU + LV were given at 1-month intervals. The trial demonstrated an overall survival (OS) benefit for the CRT group, with a median survival in the surgery-only group of 27 months versus 36 months in the CRT group. The HR for death was 1.35 (CI 95%, 1.09–1.66; $p = 0.005$). The RFS also favored the CRT group, with a median of 19 months versus 30 months; HR for relapse 1.52 (95% CI, 1.23–1.86; $p < 0.001$). The original publication had no data on histological subtypes.

A 10-year updated analysis was published in 2012 [3], and the benefit still persisted for the CRT in terms of OS with a HR of 1.32 (95% CI, 1.10–1.60; $p = 0.0046$) and for RFS with a HR of 1.51 (95% CI, 1.25–1.83; $p = 0.001$). The authors also reported an unplanned, exploratory subgroup analysis on the effect of therapy by selected patient characteristics. The results showed a trend for significant interaction in histology ($p = 0.077$), meaning that intestinal and diffuse subtypes could respond differently to CRT. The authors stated that in multivariate analysis, histology was significantly related to outcome, although no table of the multivariate analysis was given. A forest plot showed that intestinal subtype had a statistically significant benefit for OS, with a HR of approximately 1.4 (information extracted from figure); diffuse subtype had a HR of approximately 0.8, but with a confidence interval that crossed unity. The authors advise extreme caution in interpreting the results, given this was an unplanned, exploratory subanalysis and given the histologic subtype was known only in 77% of the patients (diffuse subtype accounted for 39% of the patients with known Lauren classification and 30% of the entire study).

An interesting finding of this study was that diffuse histology had better survival than intestinal histology. For example, in patients that received surgery alone, median survival was 42 months with diffuse histology versus 22 months with intestinal histology [3] (data supplement). These findings are in contrast to the general perception that diffuse-type gastric cancer carries a worse prognosis.

Although INT 0116 was a landmark trial, it was not globally accepted because of the limited lymph node dissection. Only 10% of the patients were submitted to a D2 dissection. There is debate on the benefit of a more extended lymph node dissection in gastric cancer. Some randomized studies failed to show benefit in extended dissection [4, 5], but more recent studies demonstrate better results in D2 dissection in locoregional recurrence and overall survival [6–8]. In Asia, there was a tendency to consider a D2 dissection sufficient for locoregional control.

ARTIST Trial

The ARTIST trial [9] was conducted in Korea to address the role of CRT in the setting of a D2 dissection. The trial compared adjuvant CMT versus CMT plus CRT. In the CMT arm, patients received six cycles of the XP regimen (capecitabine 1000 mg/m^2 twice daily on days 1–14; cisplatin 60 mg/m^2 on day 1 every 3 weeks). Patients assigned to the CRT arm received two cycles of XP (capecitabine 1000 mg/m^2 twice daily on days 1–14; cisplatin 60 mg/m^2 on day 1 every 3 weeks), then XRT (45 Gy at 1.8 Gy per day, 5 days per week, for 5 weeks with continuous capecitabine 825 mg/m^2 twice daily during radiotherapy), followed by two additional cycles of XP (capecitabine 1000 mg/m^2 twice daily on days 1–14; cisplatin 60 mg/m^2 on day 1 every 3 weeks). The primary endpoint was disease-free survival (DFS). For this trial, 458 patients were recruited, with 60% of patients having diffuse-subtype histology. In their first publication in 2012, the authors showed a non statistically significant difference in DFS favoring CRT. In subgroup analysis, the benefit of the CRT was statistically significant for patients with positive lymph nodes ($p = 0.035$), with a HR for DFS of 0.68 (95% CI 0.47–0.99). The authors subsequently published an update in 2015 [10] showing that there was significant interaction of both lymph node status and Lauren classification with treatment. The results demonstrated that the addition of RT to adjuvant CMT in the positive lymph node or intestinal-type subgroups significantly improved outcome.

At this point, we point out potential limitations in the sample size calculation of the ARTIST trial: The INT 0116 and the Magic trial [11] compared CRT and CMT with no adjuvant treatment. Each accrued close to 500 patients, and the HR for DFS was 1.5 in both trials. The ARTIST trial based its sample size calculation on a HR of 1.45 and recruited 458 patients. We would argue that to detect a difference in DFS between two active treatments, one should estimate a more modest HR and recruit close to twice as many patients. In addition, the ARTIST trial recruited 60% of early-stage disease patients (IB-II), resulting in fewer events (relapse or death) than was originally planned. These highlight that the overall results of the trial that demonstrated a lack of benefit of CRT in the context of adjuvant CMT could be due to a type-2 error (insufficient power to detect a difference between treatment arms).

One should also interpret with caution the results of the subgroup analyses in the INT 0116 and ARTIST trial. The positive interaction between Lauren classification and treatment suggests that intestinal and diffuse subtypes respond differently to treatment. This is different than stating that the diffuse subtype does not respond to treatment. This is illustrated by the data from the CROSS trial, which compared neoadjuvant CRT plus surgery to surgery alone in esophageal cancer [12]. The original publication showed a survival benefit favoring the CRT arm. In subgroup analysis, the benefit was statistically significant in squamous cell carcinoma (SCC) but not in adenocarcinoma. Some suggested that the results of the trial were only applicable to SCC. However, longer follow-up [13] showed that both SCC and adenocarcinoma had a statistically significant benefit with treatment, with a bigger magnitude of effect in SCC. Therefore, we advise extreme caution in the interpretation of data from subgroup analysis.

SEER Data

Stessin et al. [14] retrospectively analyzed the Surveillance, Epidemiology, and End Results (SEER) database looking at the role of adjuvant RT in the setting of diffuse gastric cancer. The authors included patients treated between 2002 and 2005 (after the publication of the INT 0116 in 2001 and before the publication of the MAGIC trial in 2006), when the expected adjuvant treatment would be CRT. They identified a total of 1889 patients with diffuse-type gastric cancer that underwent surgery and had no distant metastasis, of whom 782 received adjuvant RT and 1107 did not. Using a propensity score matching strategy, the results showed a survival benefit favoring RT, with a median survival of 30 months in the group treated with adjuvant RT versus 18 months in the group that did not receive RT ($p < 0.001$). Multivariate Cox proportional hazards regression analysis demonstrated that the addition of adjuvant RT was associated with better survival, with a HR of 0.75 (95% CI, 0.65–0.82; $p < 0.001$). Aside from the inherent limitations of the retrospective design, one important confounder was that data from CMT could not be retrieved from the SEER database. Patients in the no RT arm could have received adjuvant or perioperative CMT, despite not being standard treatment during the inclusion period. However, if a proportion of patients in the control arm did receive CMT, the results would be biased toward reducing the magnitude of benefit of RT, thus confirming that the results of this analysis are robust.

Table 7.1 summarizes selected results of studies that report the rate of diffuse subtype histology in gastric cancer.

Table 7.1 Selected results of RT in gastric cancer

Study	Type	Comparison (first standard arm)	N of Pts	Percentage diffuse(%)	OS	p-value
INT0116 (2001)	Prospective randomized	Observation vs. adjuvant CRT	556	30	Median 27 m vs. 36 m	0.005
ARTIST (2011)	Prospective randomized	Adjuvant CMT vs. CRT	458	60	5-year 73% vs. 75%	0.484
SEER (2014)	Retrospective propensity score	Adjuvant (C)RT vs. observation	1889	100	Median 30 m vs. 18 m	<0.001

N of Pts number of patients, *OS* overall survival, *CRT* chemoradiotherapy, *CMT* chemotherapy, *m* months

Meta-analysis

A Chinese meta-analysis published in 2014 [15], including 6 randomized trials comparing adjuvant CRT versus adjuvant CMT, showed that adjuvant CRT could significantly improve the 5-year DFS rate (OR 1.56, 95% CI: 1.09–2.24) and reduce the locoregional recurrence rate (OR 0.46, 95% CI: 0.32–0.67) compared with CMT, but there was no difference in 5-year OS rates (OR 1.32, 95% CI: 0.92–1.88). The authors did not have a formal statistical analysis according to histology, but almost 56% of the patients had diffuse subtype.

Patterns of Relapse

Marelli et al. conducted a multicenter longitudinal study to evaluate patterns of relapse in patients subjected to potentially curative surgery for gastric cancer with no adjuvant treatment [16]. The incidence of locoregional, hematogenous, and peritoneal recurrence were respectively 27%, 16%, and 34% in the diffuse subtype and 20%, 19%, and 9% in the intestinal subtype, respectively.

In our experience at Instituto do Câncer do Estado de São Paulo (ICESP), we retrospectively reviewed 104 patients treated with adjuvant CRT in gastric cancer [17], according to the INT0116 scheme. Most of the patients had advanced locoregional disease, with 85% having T3 or T4 tumors, 82% having positive nodes, and 42% having diffuse-type histology. The median survival was 38.3 months in intestinal subtype versus *not reached* in the diffuse subtype ($p = 0.48$). In univariate and multivariate analysis, histology was not correlated with differences in DFS or OS. Patterns of relapse were also not different, with locoregional, peritoneal, and systemic relapses of respectively 9%, 10%, and 11% for the diffuse subtype and 10%, 13%, and 13% for the intestinal subtype ($p = NS$).

The INT 0116 and ARTIST trials both showed a reduction in locoregional recurrence with CRT [3, 9], but they did not publish patterns of recurrence according to histology.

Ongoing Trials

There are currently three prospective randomized phase III trials addressing the role of RT in different scenarios of gastric cancer. All of them include both intestinal and diffuse subtypes.

The ARTIST II trial (NCT01761461) will compare adjuvant CMT versus CRT in patients with positive lymph nodes after gastrectomy plus D2 dissection. Randomization will be stratified based on histology [18].

The CRITICS trial (NCT00407186) will compare perioperative CMT with epirubicin, cisplatin, and capecitabine versus the same neoadjuvant CMT plus adjuvant CRT (45 Gy with five fractions with weekly cisplatin and daily capecitabine) in patients with gastric cancer. Randomization was stratified by histology. This trial has completed recruitment. At the initial analysis [19], OS was similar between the two groups, with a 5-year survival of 41.3% for CMT and 40.9% for CRT ($p = 0.99$). The toxicity profile was similar, except for neutropenia, where the CRT group had statistically significantly fewer events (hematological grade III or higher: 44% vs. 34%; $p = 0.01$). No subgroup analyses have been presented so far.

The TOPGEAR trial (NCT01924819) will compare preoperative CRT versus preoperative CMT for resectable gastric and gastroesophageal junction cancer. The randomization will be based on a minimization process, but patients will not be stratified by histology [20].

To the extent of our knowledge, there are no published or ongoing phase III trials addressing the role of radiation therapy specifically in diffuse-type-only gastric cancer. We acknowledge that this issue is highly controversial and that ultimately only a well-designed randomized phase III trial may settle the debate. Until then, based on the currently available data, we recommend adjuvant CRT to all patients with T2 to T4 or N+ resected gastric cancer, irrespective of histology.

Radiation Therapy Recommendations

Indications for adjuvant treatment with CRT: T2–T4 or N+.

Dose 45 Gy in 25 fractions of 1.8Gy per day, 5 fractions per week. An additional dose may be performed if margins are positive with 5.4Gy in 3 fractions of 1.8Gy per day.

Simulation Fast for 4 h before simulation computerized tomography (CT). Simulate in supine position with arms up and above the head.

Accessories Wing board or vac-fix.

Use 4D-CT to account for diaphragm motion.

Volumes of treatment Always include tumor bed, anastomosis, remaining stomach, and perigastric lymph nodes. Other locations and lymph node chains depend on primary site, T and N stage, and type of dissection.

Lymph node chains at risk according to primary site [21]:

– Gastroesophageal junction: periesophageal, mediastinal, and celiac
– Cardia and proximal: periesophageal, mediastinal, celiac, splenic, and suprapancreatic
– Body: celiac, splenic, suprapancreatic, pancreaticoduodenal, and porta hepatis

- Antrum, pylorus, and distal: celiac, suprapancreatic, pancreaticoduodenal, porta hepatis

Organs at risk Heart, lungs, liver, kidneys, and spinal cord.

Technique 3D conformal or intensity-modulated radiation therapy (IMRT); IMRT can be used to spare heart, lungs, and kidneys if organs-at-risk constraints cannot be met with 3D conformal RT. Apparently there is no difference in disease control and treatment toxicity [22, 23]. IMRT may reduce late nephrotoxicity [24].

Weekly patient evaluation during treatment looking at toxicity and early introduction of symptomatics.

Acute toxicities Fatigue, nausea, anorexia, myelosuppression (due to concomitant CMT), dyspepsia, gastritis, and ulcer.

Commonly used medicines Antiemetics as dimenhydrinate, metoclopramide or ondansetron given 1 h before treatment.

References

1. Gunderson LL, Sosin H. Adenocarcinoma of the stomach: areas of failure in a re-operation series (second or symptomatic look) clinicopathologic correlation and implications for adjuvant therapy. Int J Radiat Oncol Biol Phys. 1982;8(1):1–11.
2. Macdonald JS, Smalley SR, Benedetti J, Hundahl SA, Estes NC, Stemmermann GN, et al. Chemoradiotherapy after surgery compared with surgery alone for adenocarcinoma of the stomach or gastroesophageal junction. N Engl J Med. 2001;345(10):725–30.
3. Smalley SR, Benedetti JK, Haller DG, Hundahl SA, Estes NC, Ajani JA, et al. Updated analysis of SWOG-directed intergroup study 0116: a phase III trial of adjuvant radiochemotherapy versus observation after curative gastric cancer resection. J Clin Oncol. 2012;30(19):2327–33.
4. Dent DM, Madden MV, Price SK. Randomized comparison of R1 and R2 gastrectomy for gastric carcinoma. Br J Surg. 1988;75(2):110–2.
5. Cuschieri A, Weeden S, Fielding J, Bancewicz J, Craven J, Joypaul V, et al. Patient survival after D1 and D2 resections for gastric cancer: long-term results of the MRC randomized surgical trial. Surgical Co-operative Group Br J Cancer. 1999;79(9–10):1522–30.
6. Viste A, Svanes K, Janssen CW Jr, Maartmann-Moe H, Søreide O. Prognostic importance of radical lymphadenectomy in curative resections for gastric cancer. Eur J Surg. 1994;160(9):497–502.
7. Siewert JR, Böttcher K, Stein HJ, Roder JD. Relevant prognostic factors in gastric cancer: ten-year results of the German Gastric Cancer Study. Ann Surg. 1998;228(4):449–61.
8. Songun I, Putter H, Kranenbarg EM, Sasako M, van de Velde CJ. Surgical treatment of gastric cancer: 15-year follow-up results of the randomised nationwide Dutch D1D2 trial. Lancet Oncol. 2010;11(5):439–49.
9. Lee J, Lim DH, Kim S, Park SH, Park JO, Park YS, et al. Phase III trial comparing capecitabine plus cisplatin versus capecitabine plus cisplatin with concurrent capecitabine radiotherapy in completely resected gastric cancer with D2 lymph node dissection: the ARTIST trial. J Clin Oncol. 2012;30(3):268–73.

10. Park SH, Sohn TS, Lee J, do DH L, Hong ME, Kim KM, et al. Phase III trial to compare adjuvant chemotherapy with capecitabine and cisplatin versus concurrent chemoradiotherapy in gastric cancer: final report of the adjuvant chemoradiotherapy in stomach tumors trial, including survival and subset analyses. J Clin Oncol. 2015;33(28):3130–6.

11. Cunningham D, Allum WH, Stenning SP, Thompson JN, Van de Velde CJ, Nicolson M, et al. Perioperative chemotherapy versus surgery alone for resectable gastroesophageal cancer. N Engl J Med. 2006;355(1):11–20.

12. van Hagen P, Hulshof MC, van Lanschot JJ, Steyerberg EW, van Berge Henegouwen MI, Wijnhoven BP, et al. Preoperative chemoradiotherapy for esophageal or junctional cancer. N Engl J Med. 2012;366(22):2074–84.

13. Shapiro J, van Lanschot JJ, Hulshof MC, van Hagen P, van Berge Henegouwen MI, Wijnhoven BP, et al. Neoadjuvant chemoradiotherapy plus surgery versus surgery alone for oesophageal or junctional cancer (CROSS): long-term results of a randomised controlled trial. Lancet Oncol. 2015;16(9):1090–8.

14. Stessin AM, Sison C, Schwartz A, Ng J, Chao CK, Li B. Does adjuvant radiotherapy benefit with diffuse-type gastric cancer? Results from the surveillance, epidemiology, and end results database. Cancer. 2014;120(22):3562–8.

15. Dai Q, Jian L, Lin RJ, Wei KK, Gan LL, Deng CH, et al. Adjuvant chemoradiotherapy versus chemotherapy for gastric cancer: a meta-analysis of randomized controlled trials. J Surg Oncol. 2015;111(3):277–84.

16. Marrelli D, Roviello F, de Manzoni G, Morgagni P, Di Leo A, Saragoni L, et al. Italian research Group for Gastric Cancer. Different patterns of recurrence in gastric cancer depending on Lauren's histological type: longitudinal study. World J Surg. 2002;26(9):1160–5.

17. Vasconcelos K, Chen ATC, Hong CBC, Nakazato D, Stelko G, Hoff PMG, et al. Liver irradiation increases relapse-free survival in adjuvant gastric cancer treatment. Int J Radiat Oncol Biol Phys. 2013;87(2 Suppl 2257):S301.

18. Park SH, Lee SJ, Kim ST, Lee J, Park JO, Park YS, et al. Multicenter phase III trial of adjuvant chemoradiotherapy in stomach tumors 2 (ARTIST 2). J Clin Oncol. 2015;33(Suppl 3):TPS228.

19. Verheij M, Jansen EPM, Cats A, van Grieken NCT, Aaronson NK, Boot H, et al. A multicenter randomized phase III trial of neo-adjuvant chemotherapy followed by surgery and chemotherapy or by surgery and chemoradiotherapy in resectable gastric cancer: First results from the CRITICS study. J Clin Oncol. 2016;34(Suppl 15):4000.

20. https://www.anzctr.org.au/Trial/Registration/TrialReview.aspx?id=83497.

21. Tepper JE, Gunderson LL. Radiation treatment parameters in the adjuvant postoperative therapy of gastric cancer. Semin Radiat Oncol. 2002;12(2):187–95.

22. Ashman JB, Callister MD, Jaroszewski DE, Ross HJ, Ezzell GA, Gunderson LL. Trimodality therapy for distal esophageal/esophagogastric junction adenocarcinoma using three-dimensional conformal and intensity modulated radiotherapy. Int J Radiat Oncol Biol Phys. 2010;78(3 Suppl 2222):S303.

23. Chopra S, Agarwal A, Engineer R, Dora T, Thomas B, Sonawone S, et al. Intensity modulated radiation therapy (IMRT) is not superior to three-dimensional conformal radiation (3DCRT) for adjuvant gastric radiation: a matched pair analysis. J Cancer Res Ther. 2015;11(3):623–9.

24. Trip AK, Nijkamp J, van Tinteren H, Cats A, Boot H, Jansen EP, et al. IMRT limits nephrotoxicity after chemoradiotherapy for gastric cancer. Radiother Oncol. 2014;112(2):289–94.

Chapter 8
The Role of Chemotherapy

Guilherme Luiz Stelko Pereira and Eduardo Saadi Neto

Introduction

Systemic chemotherapy plays an important role as curative and palliative treatment for gastric cancer. As curative-intent treatment, perioperative chemotherapy, adjuvant chemotherapy, and adjuvant chemoradiation have been applied largely worldwide for locally advanced gastric cancer. As palliative treatment, chemotherapy has prolonged overall survival (OS) in different studies since the 1990s as single-agent chemotherapy, combined chemotherapy with two or three drugs, as second-line therapy, and in combination with molecular targeted agents.

Despite the well-recognized heterogeneity of gastric cancer, with different histologic subtypes described by Lauren in 1965, the effects of chemotherapy were considered independently of Lauren classification in most clinical trials, and just a few studies addressed a specific hypothesis for diffuse gastric cancer (DGC). This is more relevant once a genetic signature of DGC is described and possibly can predict different outcomes with different chemotherapy agents. In this chapter we will discuss the main clinical trials from the DGC point of view, along with a meta-analysis constructed for this purpose, some practical aspects of treatment, and perspectives of systemic treatment for DGC.

G. L. S. Pereira (✉)
Centro de Oncologia do Paraná, Curitiba, Paraná, Brazil

E. S. Neto
Hospital de Base da Faculdade de Medicina de São José do Rio Preto (FAMERP),
São José do Rio Preto (SP), Brazil

© Springer International Publishing AG, part of Springer Nature 2018
T. B. de Castria, R. S. C. Guindalini (eds.), *Diffuse Gastric Cancer*,
https://doi.org/10.1007/978-3-319-95234-5_8

Curative Chemotherapy for Diffuse Gastric Cancer

Historically in North America, adjuvant chemoradiation with fluoropyrimidine has become the standard approach to treating locally advanced gastric cancer after the Intergroup 0116 trial (INT-0116 trial), also known as the MacDonald trial, published in 2001 [1]. In Europe, the MAGIC trial, published in 2006, highlighted the perioperative chemotherapy approach, with the benefit of reducing tumor sizes, diminishing lymph node involvement, and prolonging OS [2]. Meanwhile, in Japan, where gastric surgery is traditionally recognized by the rigor of lymph node dissection, the ACTS-GC study, published by Sakuramoto et al. in 2007, demonstrated OS benefit with the adjuvant oral fluoropyrimidine agent S-1 used for 1 year [3]. Thus, in the first decade of the twenty-first century, one can say that gastric cancer patients faced different threats depending on their geographic region.

More recently, two Korean trials have investigated the benefit of adjuvant doublet fluoropyrimidine-platin chemotherapy, alone in the CLASSIC trial, or with and without chemoradiation in the ARTIST-I trial [4, 5]. These trials opened the possibility of adjuvant chemotherapy without radiotherapy, with drugs available in Western countries with a benefit in terms of OS.

Clinical Trials of Curative Chemotherapy and Diffuse Gastric Cancer

The Global Advanced/Adjuvant Stomach Tumor Research International Collaboration (GASTRIC) Group published a meta-analysis in 2010 that studied randomized clinical trials published up to 2009. Thirty-one eligible trials with 6390 patients were identified. In this meta-analysis, a statistically significant benefit was observed in terms of OS (hazard ratio [HR] 0.82; 95% confidence interval [CI] 0.76–0.90; $p < 0.001$) and disease-free survival (HR 0.82; 95% CI 0.75–0.90; $p < 0.001$) for the adjuvant chemotherapy group compared with surgery alone. It is important to highlight that no conclusion was reported regarding benefits in the diffuse subtype because most of the included clinical trials did not address this matter [6].

The INT-0116 trial has compared surgery alone with adjuvant chemotherapy with 5-fluorouracil and leucovorin, followed by chemotherapy concomitant with radiation and two more cycles of the same drugs. Most patients had a suboptimal surgery, with less than 10% of patients receiving a gastrectomy with D2 dissection. In this scenario, the protocol of adjuvant chemoradiation showed survival benefit, with a 3-year survival rate of 50% versus 41% in the surgery-alone group (HR 1,35; 95% CI 1.09–1.66; $p = 0.005$) [1].

An update of the INT-0116 trial, published in 2012, described interesting aspects regarding DGC. It reported that 169 patients, 30.2% of the studied population, were classified as having diffuse histology. In the whole population a strong persistent benefit was demonstrated from adjuvant radiochemotherapy, and it was observed that HRs were virtually unchanged from the original report. However, the interesting aspect is that subset analysis showed robust treatment benefit in most subsets, with the exception of patients with diffuse histology, who exhibited a minimal non-significant treatment effect. In women with DGC, 71 patients (12.7% of the studied population), this lack of benefit was particularly more pronounced [7].

Perioperative chemotherapy (PCT) has emerged as an important curative strategy for gastric cancer in the MAGIC trial. In this trial, patients received three cycles of ECF (epirrubicin, cisplatin, 5FU), followed by surgery, and three more cycles of ECF. Only 41% of patients had completed all six planned cycles. The original report did not describe the percentage of patients classified as having a diffuse histology [2].

The phase III French trial by FNCLCC/FFCD, published in 2011, also strengthened the benefits of PCT over surgery alone. This trial was planned to prove the benefit of PCT with cisplatin and 5FU for lower esophageal and gastroesophageal junction (GEJ) adenocarcinomas, once these represented 75% of patients in the study. An OS benefit was demonstrated for PCT, with a 38% 5-year survival rate versus 24% from surgery only (HR 0.69; 0.50–0.95, $p = 0.02$). Again, no benefit from this strategy was reported on the basis of Lauren's histologic subtype [8].

The literature contains only retrospective evidence that patients with signet-ring cell adenocarcinoma may not benefit from PCT. The FREGAT Working Group–FRENCH investigated this issue in a retrospective comparative study that included 924 patients from 19 French centers treated under a curative approach. Of those patients, 171 (18.5%) received PCT and 753 (81.5%) were treated with primary surgery. PCT was based mainly on a fluorouracil-platinum doublet or triplet regimen. The resection rate was similar in both groups (around 65%), and the median survival was shorter in the PCT group, 12.8 versus 14.0 months ($p = 0.043$). In a multivariate analysis, PCT was found to be an independent predictor of poor survival (HR = 1.4, 95% CI 1.1–1.9; $p = 0.042$). Because these conclusions were drawn on the basis of a retrospective study and not a prospective randomized trial, they should be taken with caution [9].

As described earlier, adjuvant chemotherapy is another possible curative-intent treatment for locally advanced gastric carcinoma, mainly since the ACTS-CG trial published in 2007. This trial proved the benefit of 1 year of adjuvant S-1, an oral fluoropyrimidine, in East Asian patients subjected to a D2 lymphadenectomy. In the subset analysis, the histologic subtype (undifferentiated or differentiated) was not a predictive factor. The classic Lauren classification was not applied in this study [3].

More recently, the Korean CLASSIC trial proved the benefit of adjuvant oxaliplatin and capecitabine in a similar scenario to ACTS-CG, but again the Lauren histologic classification was not applied, and it is not possible to determine the predictive potential of diffuse histology [4, 5].

Palliative Chemotherapy for Diffuse Gastric Cancer

Earlier reports published in the 1990s showed that the use of palliative systemic chemotherapy resulted in better outcomes compared with best supportive care alone [10, 11]. Although treatment options for metastatic gastric cancer (mGC) have evolved, survival is still disappointing. Several cytotoxic agents were tested in randomized clinical trials (RCTs) and are known to be active in this setting. Fluoropyrimidines, platinum agents (cisplatin and oxaliplatin), taxanes, and irinotecan are the most widely used agents [12].

The best way to combine these drugs is not a consensus and multidrug regimens; compared with monotherapy, these resulted in better response rates and OS, but with worse toxicity profile. There is no single well-established standard of care, but fluoropyrimidine-based and platinum-based combinations are the most widely used, sometimes with the addition of a third drug (docetaxel or epirubicin, for example).

Retrospective Analyses

Several retrospective trials tried to guide the choice of chemotherapy based on the histological description.

Simon Pernot et al. presented data at the 2015 ASCO annual meeting about a retrospective analysis of 45 ($N = 45$) patients, including signet-ring cell cancer (SRCC) ($N = 32$) and poorly differentiated adenocarcinoma ($N = 13$). They were treated with a combination of docetaxel, oxaliplatin, and 5-fluorouracil ("*TEFOX*" regimen) in a first-line setting. The results were interesting in terms of response rate and OS [13].

In the same context, Ali Murat Sedef et al. retrospectively analyzed 110 ($N = 110$) patients with mGC, including 17,3% histologically classified as SRCC. The chemotherapy regimens used were a combination of platinum (cisplatin) and 5-fluorouracil ("*PF*" regimen) with or without taxane ("*PFTax*" regimen). This trial failed to demonstrate a significant relation between histological types and treatment regimens, in terms of progression-free survival (PFS) and OS [14].

It is important to analyze these data with caution because they originated from a small retrospective trial.

Randomized Clinical Trials

Up to the data published in 2010 in the ToGA trial [15], the median OS with chemotherapy in first-line RCTs had never exceeded 12 months. In this study published by Bang et al., median OS reached 13.8 months by adding trastuzumab to the combination of cisplatin and fluoropyrimidine (capecitabine or 5-fluorouracil), in

Table 8.1 First-line chemotherapy – study with subgroup evaluation by histology

mGC 1st line	Study	Number of patients	Chemotherapy regimens	Stratified by histology	Primary end point	Positive trial?	Subgroup evaluation by histology?
Yung-Jue Bang et al., Lancet 2010 [15]	Phase III	594	Capecitabine *or* 5-fluoruracil + cisplatin ± trastuzumab	No (9% DGC)	Overall survival	Yes	Yes

Table 8.2 First-line chemotherapy – studies without subgroup evaluation by histology

mGC 1st line	Study	Number of patients	Chemotherapy regimens	Stratified by histology	Primary end point	Positive trial?	Subgroup evaluation by histology?
Van Cutsem et al., JCO 2014 [16]	Phase III	457	DCF vs. CF	No	Time to progression	Yes	No
Cunningham et al., NEJM 2008 [17]	Phase III	1002	EOX vs. ECX EOF vs. ECF	No	Overall survival	Yes	No
Guimbaud et al., JCO 2014 [18]	Phase III	416	ECX vs. FOLFIRI	"Yes" Linitis plastic or not	Time to progression	Yes	No
Al-Batran et al., JCO 2008 [19]	Phase III	220	FLO vs. FLP	No	Progression-free survival	No	No

JCO Journal of Clinical Oncology, *D* Docetaxel, *C* Cisplatin, *F* 5-Fluorouracil, *E* Epirubicin, *O* Oxaliplatin, *X* Capecitabine, *FLO* 5-Fluorouracil, Leucovorin, and Oxaliplatin, *FLP* 5-Fluorouracil, Leucovorin, and Cisplatin, *FOLFIRI* 5-Fluorouracil, Leucovorin, and Irinotecan

HER2-overexpressing mGC. A HER2 positivity was detected in 6.1% of DGCs (in contrast to approximately 32% in the intestinal subtype). Despite being underrepresented in the ToGA trial and subgroup analyses, no benefit has been demonstrated from adding trastuzumab to chemotherapy in DGCs (HR for OS of 1.07 [0.56–2.05]), and it is recommended that HER2 be tested in all mGCs, regardless of histology. Actually, subgroup analysis is underpowered to exclude a population of patients for the possible benefit with this specific multidrug treatment (Table 8.1).

In four other first-line RCTs, all published between 2006 and 2014, analyses of outcomes based on histology were not done [16–19]. In fact, most of them did not even mention the percentage of DGC patients enrolled. Furthermore, no subgroup analysis or specific discussion on the possible relation between chemotherapy regimens and histologic subgroups, in terms of response rate, PFS, and OS, was conducted. These trials are detailed in Table 8.2.

Table 8.3 Second-line chemotherapy

mGC 2nd line	Study	Number of patients	Chemotherapy regimens	Stratified by histology	Primary end point	Positive trial?	Subgroup evaluation by histology?
Shuichi Hironaka et al., JCO 2013 [22]	Phase III	223	Paclitaxel vs. Irinotecan	No	Overall survival	No	Yes
Jun Hun Kang et al., JCO 2012 [23]	Phase III	202	Docetaxel *or* Irinotecan vs. BSC	No	Overall survival	Yes	No

Second-Line Systemic Treatment

The choice of chemotherapy in the second line is empiric. A variety of active drugs exist, and no single regimen is considered the standard approach. Multiagent cytotoxic chemotherapy showed no advantages in terms of survival compared with monotherapy, although with increased toxicity [20–22]. Indeed, the efficacy of second-line therapy seems to be similar based on a comparison of all the active drugs, for example taxanes and irinotecan [22, 23].

However, as occurs in a first-line setting, almost none of the phase III trials in the second line included an evaluation based on distinct histological subtypes (intestinal *versus* DGC). Therefore, there are no recommendations about choosing specific cytotoxic chemotherapy based on histologic features. More details can be found in Table 8.3.

Target Therapy

The blockade of vascular endothelial growth factor receptor 2 (VEGFR-2) has emerged as an interesting treatment option in second-line mGC. In this setting, ramucirumab (a recombinant monoclonal antibody of the IgG1 class that binds to VEGFR-2) improved survival either alone or in combination with paclitaxel [24, 25].

In contrast to some trials of cytotoxic chemotherapy, the investigators from REGARD [19] and RAINBOW [25] distinguished the percentage of patients with DGC (almost 40% of all the patients enrolled in both trials). Subgroup analyses showed an improvement in outcomes across all patients, although without statistical significance for DGC in the RAINBOW trial. These are detailed in Table 8.4.

Despite these findings, there is no recommendation against the use of ramucirumab in DGC, and the outcomes in this subgroup are expected to be the same as reported in phase III trials, in terms of toxicity, survival, and response rates. More details can be found in Table 8.5.

Table 8.4 Subgroup analyses: diffuse gastric cancer (DGC) and hazard ratio (HR) for OS

VEGRF-2 blockadge	Percentage DGC (%)	HR (95%CI) for OS-DGC	HR (95%CI) for OS, intestinal subtype
REGARD trial	38–40	0. 560 (0. 366–0. 857)	1. 009 (0. 583–1. 745)
RAINBOW trial	35–40	0. 856 (0. 641–1. 145)	0. 705 (0. 534–0. 932)

JCO Journal of Clinical Oncology, *BSC* Best Supportive Care

Table 8.5 Second-line chemotherapy – targeted therapy

mGC 2nd line	Study	Number of patients	Chemotherapy regimens	Stratified by histology	Primary end point	Positive trial?	Subgroup evaluation by histology?
Fuchs CS et al.., Lancet 2014 [24]	Phase III	355	Placebo + BSC vs. Ramucirumab + BSC	No	Overall survival	Yes	Yes
Wilke H et al, Lancet Oncol., 2014 [25]	Phase III	665	Placebo + Paclitaxel vs. Ramucirumab + Paclitaxel	No	Overall survival	Yes	No

BSC Best Supportive Care

Chemotherapy and Molecular Profile of Diffuse Gastric Cancer

The potential prognostic factor based on histologic subtypes of gastric cancer is still under debate and has not yet been proven [26, 27]. It is thought that the heterogeneity in gastric cancer's biology could cause different levels of sensitivity to chemotherapy, especially between intestinal and diffuse subtypes. However, it is worth mentioning that no RCT has directly compared the efficacy of systemic chemotherapy according to Lauren's histological subtypes or molecular classification. In the metastatic scenario, the medical management of this disease is not influenced by epidemiological, histological, or anatomical features.

In vitro drug sensitivity was tested in 28 cell lines of gastric cancer in a trial conducted by Tan et al. [28]. Under classification through genomic bases, genomic diffuse (G-DIF) cell lines were more sensitive to cisplatin, while genomic intestinal (G-INT) were more sensitive to 5-fluorouracil and oxaliplatin. Although these findings suggest that molecular characterization could potentially be used to guide treatment selection, it was an early-phase and small study, which requires further validation [29].

More recently, the Cancer Genome Atlas Research Network (CGARN) analyzed the molecular characteristics of gastric adenocarcinoma, describing four different subtypes: Epstein–Barr virus (EBV) positive (9% of tumors), microsatellitte unstable tumors (22%), genomically stable tumors (20%), and tumors with chromosomal instability (50%) [30].

Most tumors classified as diffuse were concentrated in the genomically stable subtype, in which around 75% of tumors were diffuse. This subtype demonstrated infrequent targetable genetic alterations other than *RHOA* mutations and *CLDN18-ARHGAP6* or *ARHGAP26* fusions. These genes are implicated in cellular adhesion and motility, which are clearly dysregulated in diffuse-subtype tumors. Comprehensive studies are needed to confirm whether these alterations are driver mutations, and their use as targets can improve the outcomes of perioperative or adjuvant treatment in this poor prognostic subset of patients [31].

Imunotherapy

Since the advance of checkpoint inhibitors, cancer immunotherapy has been producing revolutionary results in melanoma, lung and kidney cancer, and even in early studies with many other cancers. Checkpoint inhibitors have high expectations once they target a very important hallmark of cancer cells: evasion of immune surveillance.

Recently, when used in gastric cancer, checkpoint inhibitors have been tested in early clinical trials, phase I and phase I/II in heavily pretreated patients, showing excellent results. In KEYNOTE-012, a phase Ib trial, patients with PD-L1 positive (IHC positive in >1% cells) received pembrolizumab, an anti-PD1, at a dosage of 10 mg/kg every 2 weeks. A total of 39 patients were enrolled, and an overall response rate of 22%, with a median response duration of 24 weeks, was observed [32]. In the phase II CheckMate-032, nivolumab, another anti-PD1, was tested in pretreated gastric cancer patients regardless of PD-L1 status. The confirmed objective response rate among 59 patients reached 14%, and 36% of patients survived to 1 year [33]. These early trials did not discriminate between diffuse and nondiffuse tumors. In 2016, a global phase III trial with pembrolizumab in the first-line setting, alone or in combination with chemotherapy, was launched, and its final results are expected to be published in 2018.

Of note, DGC represents around 25% of the EBV positive tumor subtype described by the Cancer Genome Atlas Research Network. This subtype is characterized by a significant increase in PD-L1 expression and, as consequence, is a good candidate for immune checkpoint inhibitor studies. The microsatellite unstable (MSI) subtype harbors a high mutation load and is also an interesting candidate for immunotherapy, but the frequency of DGC is only around 10% in the MSI subtype [30].

Conclusion

DGC has specific clinical, epidemiological, and pathological characteristics, though there is no strong evidence on which to base a choice of systemic therapy according to the histological classification, in either a curative or palliative setting. On a few clinical trials have been designed specifically for DGC, and most of the pivotal trials have not even reported results according to Lauren's classification. In an adjuvant setting, it is probable that women with a diffuse histology would not benefit from chemoradiation with 5FU as performed in the INT-0116 trial, and combination adjuvant chemotherapy as in the CLASSIC trial appears to be a better option. In a metastatic setting, a low frequency of HER-2 superexpression precludes the use of trastuzumab for the vast majority of patients. Although a small study suggested a benefit from choosing cisplatin for tumors with a diffuse genetic signature, this information requires further prospective validation. The DIGEST trial for DGC fails to prove the superiority of S1 over regular doublet chemotherapy. Therefore, it is recommended that diffuse mGC, including SRCC histology, be treated with the available regimens of systemic chemotherapy, either in first or in subsequent lines, and target therapy (antibodies targeting VEGRF-2 or HER2), if indicated, regardless of Lauren classification.

Furthermore, the new molecular classification of gastric cancer described earlier may lead to practical applications, including the choice of immunotherapy for specific genetic signatures of gastric cancer. In the future, this may prove to be an adequate tool, better than the histopathological classification currently available, to individualize treatment for gastric cancer patients in daily practice.

References

1. Macdonald JS, Smalley SR, Benedetti J, Hundahl SA, Estes NC, Stemmermann GN, et al. Chemoradiotherapy after surgery compared with surgery alone for adenocarcinoma of the stomach or gastroesophageal junction. N Engl J Med. 2001;345:725–30.
2. Cunningham D, Allum WH, Stenning SP, Thompson JN, Van de Velde CJ, Nicolson M, et al. Perioperative chemotherapy versus surgery alone for Resectable gastroesophageal Cancer. N Engl J Med. 2006;355:11–20.
3. Sakuramoto S, Sasako M, Yamaguchi T, Kinoshita T, Fujii M, Nashimoto A, et al. Adjuvant chemotherapy for gastric Cancer with S-1, an oral Fluoropyrimidine. N Engl J Med. 2007;357:1810–20.
4. Bang YJ, Kim YW, Yang HK, Chung HC, Park YK, Lee KH, et al. Adjuvant capecitabine and oxaliplatin for gastric cancer after D2 gastrectomy (CLASSIC): a phase 3 open-label, randomised controlled trial. Lancet. 2012;379:315–21.
5. Park SH, Sohn TS, Lee J, Lim DH, Hong ME, Kim KM, et al. Phase III trial to compare adjuvant chemotherapy with Capecitabine and cisplatin versus concurrent Chemoradiotherapy in gastric Cancer: final report of the adjuvant Chemoradiotherapy in stomach tumors trial, including survival and subset analyses. J Clin Oncol. 2015;33(28):3130–6.

6. GASTRIC Group, Paoletti X, Oba K, Burzykowski T, Michiels S, Ohashi Y, et al. Benefit of adjuvant chemotherapy for resectable gastric cancer: a meta-analysis. JAMA. 2010;303(17):1729–37.
7. Smalley SR, Benedetti JK, Haller DG, Hundahl SA, Estes NC, Ajani JA, et al. Updated analysis of SWOG-directed intergroup study 0116: a phase III trial of adjuvant Radiochemotherapy versus observation after curative gastric Cancer resection. J Clin Oncol. 2012;19:2327–33.
8. Ychou M, Boige V, Pignon JP, Conroy T, Bouché O, Lebreton G, et al. Perioperative chemotherapy compared with surgery alone for resectable gastroesophageal adenocarcinoma: an FNCLCC and FFCD multicenter phase III trial. J Clin Oncol. 2011;29(13):1715–21.
9. Messager M, Lefevre JH, Pichot-Delahaye V, Souadka A, Piessen G, Mariette C, et al. The impact of perioperative chemotherapy on survival in patients with gastric signet ring cell adenocarcinoma: a multicenter comparative study. Ann Surg. 2011;254(5):684–93.
10. Pyrhönen S, Kuitunen T, Nyandoto P, Kouri M. Randomised comparison of fluorouracil, epidoxorubicin and methotrexate (FEMTX) plus supportive care versus supportive care alone in patients with non-resectable gastric cancer. Br J Cancer. 1995;71(3):587–91.
11. Glimelius B, Ekström K, Hoffman K, Graf W, Sjödén PO, et al. Randomized comparison between chemotherapy plus best supportive care with best supportive care in advanced gastric cancer. Ann Oncol. 1997;8(2):163–8.
12. Wagner AD, Grothe W, Haerting J, Kleber G, Grothey A, Fleig WE. Chemotherapy in advanced gastric Cancer: a systematic review and meta-analysis based on aggregate data. J Clin Oncol. 2006;24:2903–9.
13. Pernot S, Dubreuil O, Tougeron D, Soudan D, Bachet JB, Lepère C, et al. Docetaxel, 5FU, oxaliplatin (TEFOX) in 1st line treatment of signet ring cell and/or poorly differentiated gastric adenocarcinoma: a retrospective study of AGEO. J Clin Oncol. 2015;33(15_suppl):e15048.
14. Sedef AM, Köse F, Sümbül AT, Doğan Ö, Beşen AA, Tatlı AM, et al. Patients with distal intestinal gastric cancer have superior outcome with addition of taxanes to combination chemotherapy, while proximal intestinal and diffuse gastric cancers do not: does biology and location predict chemotherapy benefit? Med Oncol. 2015;32:18.
15. Bang YJ, Van Cutsem E, Feyereislova A, Chung HC, Shen L, Sawaki A, et al. Trastuzumab in combination with chemotherapy versus chemotherapy alone for treatment of HER2-positive advanced gastric or gastro-oesophageal junction cancer (ToGA): a phase 3, open-label, randomized controlled trial. Lancet. 2010;376:687–97.
16. Van Cutsem E, Moiseyenko VM, Tjulandin S, Majlis A, Constenla M, Boni C, et al. Phase III study of docetaxel and cisplatin plus fluorouracil compared with cisplatin and fluorouracil as first-line therapy for advanced gastric Cancer: a report of the V325 study group. J Clin Oncol. 2006;24:4991–7.
17. Cunningham D, Starling N, Rao S, Iveson T, Nicolson M, Coxon F, et al. Capecitabine and Oxaliplatin for advanced Esophagogastric Cancer. N Engl J Med. 2008;358:36–46.
18. Guimbaud R, Louvet C, Ries P, Ychou M, Maillard E, André T, et al. Prospective, randomized, multicenter, phase III study of Fluorouracil, Leucovorin, and irinotecan versus Epirubicin, cisplatin, and Capecitabine in advanced gastric adenocarcinoma: a French intergroup (Fédération francophone de Cancérologie digestive, Fédération Nationale des Centres de Lutte Contre le Cancer, and Groupe Coopérateur Multidisciplinaire en Oncologie) study. J Clin Oncol. 2014;32:3520–6.
19. Al-Batran SE, Hartmann JT, Probst S, Schmalenberg H, Hollerbach S, Hofheinz R, et al. Phase III trial in metastatic gastroesophageal adenocarcinoma with fluorouracil, Leucovorin plus either Oxaliplatin or cisplatin: a study of the Arbeitsgemeinschaft Internistische Onkologie. J Clin Oncol. 2016;26:1435–42.
20. Higuchi K, Tanabe S, Shimada K, Hosaka H, Sasaki E, Nakayama N, et al. Biweekly irinotecan plus cisplatin versus irinotecan alone as second-line treatment for advanced gastric cancer: a randomised phase III trial (TCOG GI-0801/BIRIP trial). Eur J Cancer. 2014;50(8):1437–45.

21. Sym SJ, Hong J, Park J, Cho EK, Lee JH, Park YH, et al. A randomized phase II study of biweekly irinotecan monotherapy or a combination of irinotecan plus 5-fluorouracil/leucovorin (mFOLFIRI) in patients with metastatic gastric adenocarcinoma refractory to or progressive after first-line chemotherapy. Cancer Chemother Pharmacol. 2013;71(2):481–8.
22. Hironaka S, Ueda S, Yasui H, Nishina T, Tsuda M, Tsumura T, et al. Randomized, open-label, phase III study comparing irinotecan with paclitaxel in patients with advanced gastric Cancer without severe peritoneal metastasis after failure of prior combination chemotherapy using Fluoropyrimidine plus platinum: WJOG 4007 trial. J Clin Oncol. 2013;31:4438–44.
23. Kang JH, Lee SI, Lim DH, Park KW, Oh SY, Kwon HC, et al. Salvage chemotherapy for pretreated gastric cancer: a randomized phase III trial comparing chemotherapy plus best supportive care with best Sspportive care alone. J Clin Oncol. 2012;30:1513–8.
24. Fuchs CS, Tomasek J, Yong CJ, Dumitru F, Passalacqua R, Goswami C, et al. Ramucirumab plus paclitaxel versus placebo plus paclitaxel in patients with previously treated advanced gastric or gastro-oesophageal junction adenocarcinoma (REGARD): a double-blind, randomized phase 3 trial. Lancet. 2014;383:31–9.
25. Wilke H, Muro K, Van Cutsem E, Oh SC, Bodoky G, Shimada Y, et al. Ramucirumab plus paclitaxel versus placebo plus paclitaxel in patients with previously treated advanced gastric or gastro-oesophageal junction adenocarcinoma (RAINBOW): a double-blind, randomised phase 3 trial. Lancet Oncol. 2014;15(11):1224–35.
26. Wu CW, Hsieh MC, Lo SS, Tsay SH, Li AF, Lui WY, et al. Prognostic indicators for survival after curative resection for patients with carcinoma of the stomach. Dig Dis Sci. 1997;42:1265–9.
27. Liu L, Wang ZW, Ji J, Zhang JN, Yan M, Zhang J, et al. A cohort study and meta-analysis between histopathological classification and prognosis of gastric carcinoma. Anti Cancer Agents Med Chem. 2013;13(2):227–34.
28. Bittoni A, Scartozzi M, Giampieri R, Faloppi L, Bianconi M, Mandolesi A, et al. Clinical evidence for three distinct gastric cancer subtypes:time for a new approach. PLoS One. 2013;8:e78544.
29. Tan IB, Ivanova T, Lim KH, Ong CW, Deng N, Lee J, et al. Intrinsic subtypes of Gastric Cancer, based on gene expression pattern, predict survival and respond differently to chemotherapy. Gastroenterology. 2011;141(2):476–85.
30. Cancer Genome Atlas Research Network. Comprehensive molecular characterization of gastric adenocarcinoma. Nature. 2014;513(7517):202–9.
31. Choi AH, Kim J, Chao J. Perioperative chemotherapy for resectable gastric cancer: MAGIC and beyond. World J Gastroenterol. 2015;21(24):7343–8.
32. Muro K, Chung HC, Shankaran V, Geva R, Catenacci D, Gupta S, et al. Pembrolizumab for patients with PD-L1-positive advanced gastric cancer (KEYNOTE-012): a multicentre, open-label, phase 1b trial. The Lancet Oncol. 2016;17(60):717–6.
33. Le DT, Bendell JC, Calvo E, Kim JW, Ascierto PA, Sharma P, et al. Safety and activity of nivolumab monotherapy in advanced and metastatic (A/M) gastric or gastroesophageal junction cancer (GC/GEC): Results from the CheckMate-032 study. J Clin Oncol. 2016;34(4_suppl):6.

Index

© Springer International Publishing AG, part of Springer Nature 2018
T. B. de Castria, R. S. C. Guindalini (eds.), *Diffuse Gastric Cancer*,
https://doi.org/10.1007/978-3-319-95234-5

Printed in the United States
By Bookmasters